Disabled, Female, and Proud!

Disabled, Female, and <u>Proud</u>!

Stories of Ten Women with Disabilities

by Harilyn Rousso

with Susan Gushee O'Malley and Mary Severance
photographs by Flo Fox

Bergin & Garvey
Westport, Connecticut • London

Library of Congress Cataloging-in-Publication Data

Rousso, Harilyn, 1946-
     Disabled, female, and proud! : stories of ten women with
disabilities / by Harilyn Rousso, with Susan Gushee O'Malley and
Mary Severance ; photographs by Flo Fox.—1st ed., 2nd printing.
     p.   cm.
     Reprint. Originally published: Boston, MA: Exceptional Parent
Press, 1988.
     Includes bibliographical references (131-134).
     Contents: Hermina Jackson—Adrienne Asch—Barbara Cole-Appel—
Nansie Sharpless—Linda O. Young—Dorothy Wainer—Geri
Strong—Alice Crespo—Connie Panzarino—Carol Ann Roberson.
     ISBN 0-89789-358-1 (pbk. : alk. paper)
     1. Handicapped women—United States—Biography.   I. O'Malley,
Susan Gushee, 1942-   .   II. Severance, Mary.   III. Title.
HV1569.3.W65R68   1993
362.4'082—dc20   93-26049

Library of Congress Catalog Card Number: 93-26049
ISBN: 0-89789-358-1

First published in 1988
Reprinted in 1993

Bergin & Garvey, 88 Post Road West, Westport, CT 06881
An imprint of Greenwood Publishing Group, Inc.

Printed in the United States of America

The paper used in this book complies with the
Permanent Paper Standard issued by the National
Information Standards Organization (Z39.48-1984).

10 9 8 7 6 5 4 3 2 1

TABLE OF CONTENTS

ACKNOWLEDGMENTS

My deepest thanks go to the YWCA of the City of New York for sponsoring the Networking Project for Disabled Women and Girls, and for creating a supportive environment in which all this work was possible. I also want to thank my dear friend Linda Nessel for encouraging me to translate my ideas about the needs of disabled women and girls into actions. I would not have undertaken this book or the Networking Project without her persistent support and inspiration.

My heartfelt appreciation goes to the ten women profiled in this book for so freely giving their time and sharing their lives. Through seemingly endless interviews, photograph sessions, reviews of drafts, and last minute details, they maintained their commitment, their sense of humor, and their hope that younger generations of disabled women will have an easier road to a satisfying life as the result of our collective efforts.

In writing this book, I was fortunate to have the invaluable assistance of Susan Gushee O'Malley, who worked extensively on the profiles of Adrienne Asch, Barbara Cole-Appel, Alice Crespo, Connie Panzarino, Carol Ann Roberson, Geri Strong, and Dorothy Wainer; and Mary Severance, who helped research and write the remaining three profiles and review the entire manuscript. I am grateful to them both.

My thanks also go to Moira Griffin for her help in conducting some of the early research; to Katinka Neuhof for her suggestions about the bibliography; to Gene Brown for his excellent editorial help; and to Linda Marks and Claire Harnan for their abundant moral support.

Flo Fox is to be congratulated for her perseverance in tracking down and photographing most of the women who appear in this book, despite their hectic schedules; a talented artist and role model herself, she captured their spirit. Bettye Lane, Geri Tommasino and Kyle Bajakian also contributed photographs. I thank them for their fine work.

It is a particular pleasure for me that *Exceptional Parent* is the publisher of this book. My very first published article appeared in that magazine, in December 1981. I have warm feelings and much respect for the editors and am grateful for their repeated displays of confidence in my work. I am delighted to have had the opportunity to work again with Ellen Herman in preparing this manuscript for publication and thank her for her expert assistance.

This book was partially funded by grants from the Frances L. and Edwin L. Cummings Memorial Fund, the J.M. Foundation, the New York Community Trust, and the U.S. Department of Education, under the auspices of the Women's Educational Equity Act. I appreciate their support. Opinions expressed in the text do not necessarily reflect the positions or policies of these funding sources, and no official endorsement should be inferred.

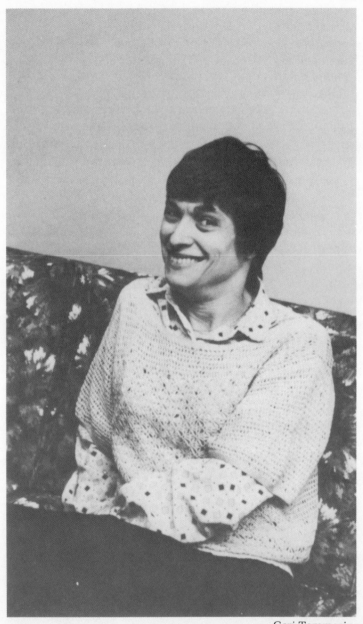

Geri Tommasino

INTRODUCTION

by Harilyn Rousso

This book is part of my work with the Networking Project for Disabled Women and Girls, a program sponsored by the YWCA of the City of New York that provides disabled women and girls with opportunities to meet and share experiences. The idea for both the book and the Networking Project came from my own personal experiences struggling with my identity as a disabled woman.

I grew up with a disability, cerebral palsy. When I was growing up, I did not know any disabled children or adults, partly because I attended regular public schools in which I was the only disabled student. But I also tried to stay away from other disabled people, to avoid them. My disability had caused me so many painful experiences—people teasing, staring, disliking me because I happened to look a bit different and do things somewhat differently—that I did not

want to be associated with others who had the very charac-
teristic which had caused me such distress. As a teenager, I
spent a lot of time covering up my physical differences, trying
to "pass" for non-disabled. At that time, I didn't realize that
it was society's prejudices against people with disabilities
rather than the disability itself that was the problem. It never
occurred to me that there might be disabled people out there
who were interesting, smart, attractive, funny, successful. At
least I had never met any.

When I was about twenty-two, I had an unexpected, important experience. I worked one summer for a prominent
woman economist who happened to have cerebral palsy. I
can't tell you my surprise when I met her at the job interview.
It was a bit like looking at myself in the mirror. Betty had a
powerful effect on me. I was impressed that a woman with
cerebral palsy, not a very socially acceptable disability in our
culture, could become so successful in her career, particularly in a "man's field," anti-trust economics.

I was even more impressed that she was married. One
of the myths in our society about disabled women is that we
are asexual, incapable of leading socially and sexually fulfill-
ing lives. When I was growing up, my parents and I accepted
this myth without question. We simply assumed that because
I had a disability, I could not date, find a partner, or have
children. As a teenager and young adult, I put aside any hope
of a social life and concentrated on my studies. It never occurred to me that I had any alternative, that I could have *both*
a career and a romantic life. Betty's lifestyle, her successful
marriage to an interesting, dynamic man made me question
for the first time the negative assumptions I had made about
my social potential. She planted the seeds of positive possibilities, which began blossoming in my mid-twenties, when
I explored the social scene for the first time. Dating can be difficult for a woman with a disability; my non-disabled women

friends tell me it can be difficult for a woman without a disability. But knowing that another woman with a disability similar to my own had gone out there and done well helped me to take the risks I needed to begin. Myths about disabled women also influenced my decision to become a psychiatric social worker and psychotherapist. Our culture tends to define female sexuality and womanhood in terms of physical perfection and beauty. We are perceived as more "womanly" the closer we come to meeting Madison Avenue or Hollywood standards of beauty. As a young girl with a disability, I felt quite far removed from those standards, and as a result I did not feel very confident about myself as a woman. When I was in college, I majored in economics, but after college, I switched to social work. I made that decision for many reasons, but an important one was my desire to identify and be identified with a "woman's profession." This choice enabled me to feel more solid as a woman. I did not yet recognize that having a disability is quite compatible with being female, and that defining womanhood in terms of physical perfection is both narrow and narrow-minded. Although I love my work, I wish now that as a young person I had felt freer to explore a broader range of careers, including those not traditionally associated with women.

Unfortunately, choosing my career did not end my struggle with societal stereotypes about disabled women. It was just the beginning. After completing a masters degree in social work, I went on for advanced training in psychotherapy. I had been enrolled for about a year in a psychotherapy training institute when I was asked to leave the school because some of the teachers did not think that a person with my disability should become a psychotherapist. They claimed that the disability would be too stressful for clinic patients to handle and suggested that I consider another career. This was a shocking and devastating experience, the most blatant example of discrimination I had ever faced. As a coping strategy, I sought out other therapists with disabilities to find out how they had survived. Many had faced experiences similar to my own. These therapists were powerful influences, offering support, concrete tactics for fighting prejudice, and the strength to persist. (Incidentally, I wound up suing the institute, which was a tremendously empowering experience and was responsible for changing me into a disability rights activist.)

As my story indicates, meeting other people, particularly other women, with disabilities had an important effect on me as an adult. I suspect it would have had even a more profound effect had I been younger, in earlier stages of making major life choices.

Unfortunately, this type of book did not exist when I was growing up, some forty years ago. At that time, there was no women's movement and no disability rights movement. Disabled women had not yet begun to organize on their own behalf or for the benefit of younger generations of women.

In 1984, I approached the YWCA of the City of New York and asked for its support in sponsoring a unique program that would provide disabled adolescent girls in the community with the very type of experience I had missed when I was growing up: opportunities to meet older disabled women leading interesting, satisfying lives who could help counteract stereotypes about being disabled and female. The YWCA was extremely enthusiastic and helped me to raise funds for the project. As a result, the Networking Project for Disabled Women and Girls was born. Through this program, disabled women and girls get together at conferences, workshops, the women's workplaces, one-to-one encounters, and special events celebrating the accomplishments of disabled women, such as an art exhibit featuring disabled women artists. The participants talk openly about many different topics, from jobs to relationships to sex. Similar programs are now being developed in other cities, including Albany, Los Angeles, Philadelphia, Pittsburgh, Spokane, and Westchester County. If you would like to find out whether a Networking Project exists in your area, or if you would like to help set one up, contact me at the address listed in the back of the book under "Resources Developed by the Networking Project."

This book is one of several resources developed by the Networking Project. It is another way to help young women with disabilities learn about the experiences of older disabled women who have "been there."

I am delighted to introduce the ten women with disabilities who are profiled in this book. I think you will find them an exciting group of women. They offer new ideas about work, relationships, lifestyles, and other areas of life that you might want to consider as you start thinking about your own future.

I have deliberately chosen women who have made different types of life choices. For example, some work in the creative arts while others work in math and science; some work in the business world while still others work in the human services.

There are women who have partners and others who are single; women who have children, and others who do not. Some of the women have been intensely involved in the disability rights, civil rights, and/or women's movements; for others, political activism has been less important. These women have a variety of opinions on such questions as how to handle disability with prospective employers and whether and how to ask for assistance and accommodations on-the-job. They differ on whether they prefer disabled or non-disabled partners, and whether they want to and feel able to raise children.

By presenting these diverse women, I hope to show that you do not have to be or become any one thing because you are a women or because you have a disability. There are, in fact, a range of possibilities from which you can choose. There is also a network of adult disabled women leading productive, satisfying lives, and we are eager to serve as a support for you as you make your way in a world that does not always recognize your potential.

As women with disabilities, we face a double set of prejudices, based on gender *and* disability. In talking about my own life experiences, I have already mentioned how the world too often sees us in terms of stereotypes: childlike, dependent, incompetent, asexual, unable to take on the roles of worker, sexual partner, or mother. Sometimes even people who know us well and love us—like family, teachers, and friends—accept these distorted images. As a result, we may become confused about who we are and who we can become.

This is where contact with successful adult women with disabilities can be most helpful. To some degree, all of the women profiled in this book have faced these same prejudices about their potential at school, at work, or in their social lives. But they have found ways to make satisfying choices for themselves despite the barriers, and they invite you to draw upon their experiences to do the same. They encourage you to make choices which go beyond society's stereotypes and reflect your own unique talents, interests, and dreams, while at the same time taking into account your real limitations and needs.

As I described, it took me a long time to "come out of the closet" as a disabled woman and feel perfectly all right about myself, disability and all. What I hope most for you is that as the result of meeting the women in this book and hearing their stories, you will feel that you neither have to avoid disability issues nor dwell on them. Rather, you can put your disability into perspective as one acceptable, O.K. part of yourself and your experience. Hopefully, your generation can feel disabled, female, *and* proud!

Harilyn Rousso, October 1987

Stories

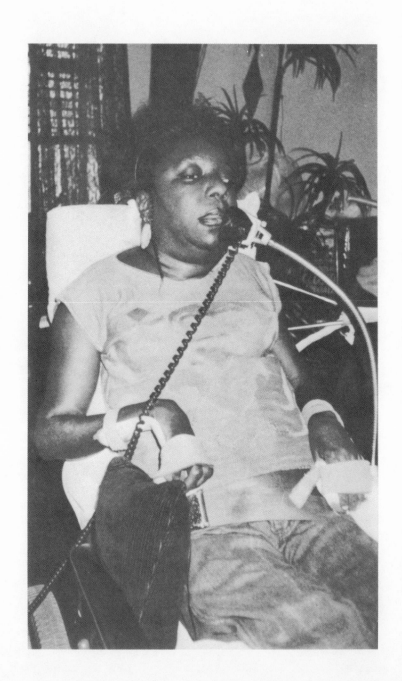

1

Hermina Jackson

COMMUNITY ACTIVIST

"I like making things happen and I like seeing results. I like one-to-one contact with people—seeing things develop. My main interest is bringing information to the black community, because we don't have it—especially not black people with disabilities. We don't have access to things like getting a wheelchair or to health and other needed services. That's my main thing."

Hermina Jackson is a community activist. She is also an energetic forty-three-year-old woman who is quadriplegic and lives in her own apartment in Brooklyn, New York. She has home care attendants and she uses a motorized wheelchair with a mouthstick to get around and do most of her day-to-day work—a lot of talking on the telephone to make contacts in the community, plan events, and exchange information. At the time of this interview, Hermina was figuring out how to use her new VCR while at the same time counseling someone over the telephone.

Hermina loves everything about what she does, except, as she says, "I don't get paid for it!" She belongs to many organizations, including Disabled In Action, Independent Living for the Handicapped of Brooklyn, the Center for Independence of the Disabled of New York, Concepts for Independent Living, the Black United Front, and the Networking Project for Disabled Women and Girls.

> Basically, whatever organization I'm involved with, I'm like a sponge. I'm always there to absorb as much information as I can, so I can take it back and give it to the community.

As a member of the Black United Front, Hermina is interested in the issues and needs of women, especially women with disabilities. She aims not only to get information for women with disabilities (information about benefits, legal rights, and practical things like where to look for a good wheelchair), but to educate the community about disabled women and what they need and how they feel. "The Black United Front is a grassroots organization developed by African descendants," she says. "It has chapters in several states in addition to New York, and it aims to strengthen and unite the black community." At the moment, she is planning for a conference at which she will show a videotape about a black South African woman who is blind. It was made when the woman recently visited the United States for a protest against the South African Government's policy of apartheid— segregation and discrimination against black people in that country. Hermina plans to lead a discussion about the videotape and issues related to it. This way, she can combine disability with other important concerns, and provide information on many issues at one meeting.

Hermina's skills in advocating (speaking out for groups of people who are usually ignored and neglected by society in general) and networking (bringing together people with different kinds of resources, like a person with a van and a person who needs that van to get around) to solve problems for people in her community developed during her teenage years, when she was living in Goldwater Memorial Hospital. She lived in the hospital for seventeen years, from age thirteen when she had the accident that led to her becoming quadriplegic until she left in 1975 at age thirty to live on her own in Brooklyn. Hermina received her high school diploma through home instruction and then attended the New School for Social Research and Queensborough Community College (starting in 1973, when she was twenty-eight years old), to be trained as a liaison between social workers and their clients. A liaison is a go-between, a person who helps two people (in this case, a client and a social worker) come together and understand each other. For example, a liaison may speak with the parents of a child in a day care center to build trust and get needed information about a family problem when the parents are reluctant to talk with the staff social worker. She decided to be a liaison because it meant fewer years in school than social workers need, and she "didn't want to be in school for a long time."

However, after she spent a semester in a training internship, Hermina decided that the job of liaison was not suited to her. She says that the issue of disability benefits was one factor in her decision to work as a volunteer. She did not want to risk losing her home attendant care, since the government would not continue to cover the cost of an attendant once she had a paying job and she knew she would not be able to afford the expense on her own. But there were other reasons for her choice. As a liaison, she was restricted to being a go-between for two other people, and she felt her creativity was not fully utilized. She also believed that the limited amount of time she had for each client, and the limited options she could present to clients, made the job seem like an "assembly line" process, impersonal and ineffective. She came to feel that she was working for the very system that she wanted to fight. She wanted to help people find options and solutions to their problems in their own communities, instead of forcing them to rely on a system that did not meet their needs.

Hermina likes the flexibility of working on her own, and not at a 9 to 5 job five days a week.

Now I can do things at my own pace, and I can work one-on-one, and see a project develop. I have a schedule set out for myself, with deadlines and things, but I leave room for myself.

She makes her transportation arrangements through networking with many different people who she meets in her community work, and thus does not rely on one company or person all the time. She tells almost everyone she meets about her transportation needs, and comes up with a good number of options that way. "Just this morning," she said, "I met someone at a meeting who has a van." Often, the organizations she works with reimburse her for the cost of her round trips to meetings and events.

Hermina's years in the hospital led her to the conclusion that the first skill she had to have was self-advocacy—speaking up for her rights and getting what she needed for herself. She thinks that this is especially important for people with disabilities.

If you don't learn to take charge of your life, if you don't talk to people, you won't find out how to get anything you need. If you want to get anywhere, you have to fight.

While living in the hospital, she visited her family in Harlem and they visited her quite often, but the hospital became her home. She says it was hard in the beginning, but as she got older, she came to see living away from home as an advantage.

In the hospital I was always involved with something. I was among my peers. Especially when you get to be a teenager, you need friends with similar interests, who are in your same situation. You go through all those feelings, about dating and sexuality, and you can do it together.

Hermina and a group of other young people in the hospital learned to take control of their lives when they decided to campaign for their own ward. In the beginning, about twelve young people got to know each other, planned some trips and activities together, and met informally to talk about the things they were going through—from their social lives and medical issues, to preparing for the "real world." Eventually, they decided that they wanted to live together in the same ward, with nurses, doctors, and therapists who "would understand our needs and how young people felt about things." They wanted help in preparing to leave the hospital, too.

It took about two years, but the hospital finally agreed to their demands.

After we got the ward, it was like a boarding school. On Sundays, everybody would have company and they would bring all kinds of food. When everyone went home, we would share all the food with each other.

She also thinks that living away from home helped her deal with her mother's overprotectiveness. Her mother worried whenever Hermina went on trips outside the hospital on her own, so Hermina "did things anyway, and told her afterward." In time, her mother stopped worrying so much.

Hermina did not leave the hospital until she was sure she was ready.

I was preparing myself for about a year. We [the group of young people in the ward] helped each other; we networked. The ones that were outside would tell you: "If you need this, then you call this person." That's what we do now for people still inside, and those of us who are outside continue to help one another.

The biggest change in living on her own was making all the choices in her everyday life, big and small.

That was something to get used to—making decisions. Simple things like when you want to eat and what; what medication to take; how you should place yourself on a schedule.

Now that she lives in her own apartment, Hermina looks back with wonder at how restrictive life was in the hospital. When she went back recently to see a doctor and have some tests, she remembers thinking: "I can't believe this place is so dead!"

She is still in touch with many of the others who were in her ward, and is planning to hold a big reunion in the near future, "with t-shirts and everything."

When she was sixteen, Hermina met a man who wanted very much to marry her. Her mother, she says, "was for it— she thought I'd need someone to take care of me," but she did not push her daughter. Hermina did not want to get married. She sees now that she was afraid of becoming too dependent on this man.

> At that time, I felt that he wouldn't stay with me. I was afraid...he was sincere, he was very sincere, but I didn't think he was. Later on in life, I realized that it was the best thing. I would never have grown. He was so protective, he would have done everything for us, taken care of too many things. If I had married him, I would never have become the woman I am now.

Hermina has had several long-term relationships with men, but has never wanted to get married.

> Relationships are fine. But I am afraid of the institution of marriage. I need to be my own woman. I don't think I could share so much—I need to know that I always have someplace else to go, like my own apartment.

Even though she never had a desire to get married, or to have children, Hermina has a strong belief in family. Her brothers and sisters, nieces, and a nephew all live in the New York area, and she sees them regularly. They are an important part of her life, and always have been. She also has an adopted daughter of her own, a young woman from the neighborhood with some personal problems who began to confide in Hermina and at age sixteen came to live with her. Hermina says that she has several "adopted" children from her community, but that this daughter is closest to her. Her daughter, now twenty-six, recently gave birth to her second child, and lives in the Bronx; she frequently travels back and forth with her children to visit Hermina.

Hermina's commitment to helping people has never changed. She says that you need confidence in yourself and a real love for people to succeed as a community activist.

> You need to work hard for yourself first before you can do anything for others. You need to advocate for your own needs. You can't get anything you don't know how to get. If I sit here and say, "well, you do it this way," you still won't know unless you actually *do* it yourself.

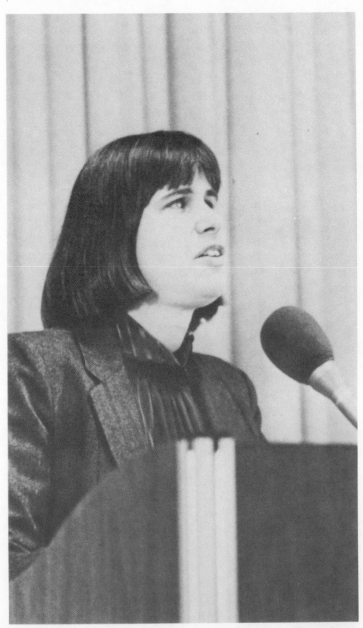

Bettye Lane

2

Adrienne Asch

CIVIL RIGHTS INVESTIGATOR

Adrienne: Since you got your job back as middle
manager of your brokerage house,
what have you been doing?

Manager: I sit here in my office, collect my pay,
and do nothing.

Adrienne: How do you feel about this?

Manager: I don't dare complain because I'm
getting paid.

Adrienne Asch is a civil rights investigator for the New York State Division of Human Rights who is blind. The young black man she was questioning had been fired despite good evaluations. The Division found that he had been discriminated against because of his race and ordered the brokerage firm where he had been working to rehire him. But since his return he had been given no responsibilities and had been improperly paid. As a result of Adrienne's investigation, his company restored his full salary and assigned him suitable work duties.

A civil rights investigator examines complaints of discrimination based on race, creed, religion, sex, disability, age, marital status, and national origin. Adrienne interviews both employers who are charged with discriminating and employees who claim to have been discriminated against. She reads documents, makes job site visits, and writes reports about what she has learned. A civil rights investigator has to be good at working with details, and able to work with a wide variety of people, some of whom she may not like. According to Adrienne, her job involves detective work.

> You've got to sniff out when people are lying and get people who are not necessarily of your race, gender, or class to tell you things and trust you, or not trust you and be unguarded enough to reveal themselves. You're dealing with a lot of data quickly and lots of cases at one time. You can't spend all of the time that any single case needs. When you're in the middle of one case, a crisis may happen in another, and if you can't shift from one topic to another very quickly, you'll go nuts. But civil rights is a wonderful field because you're dealing with an important law.

Adrienne was offered the job of civil rights investigator while she was working as a lobbyist for the New York State Human Rights Law. A lobbyist tries to convince legislators that a bill should or should not be passed and become a law. She got into lobbying when she was turned down for many jobs after she graduated from college in 1969. One rejection particularly angered her.

I applied for a job helping set up concerts at Lincoln Center in their education program. The reason I was exceptionally well qualified was I had been manager of a choir and orchestra in New Jersey, setting up concerts, running the organization, writing publicity material, getting arts council grants. I knew much more than most beginning people about how to set up concerts in public schools. And I even had a letter of reference from a conductor who had conducted at Lincoln Center.

I got an interview with the personnel person and he said, "If you had put that you were blind on your resume, I would never let you in, but here you are." [Adrienne never includes information about her disability on her resume.] He said that I had persuaded him that I could probably do the job so he called up the person I would be working with and she refused to interview me. I said, "I'm not leaving until she interviews me; she doesn't have to give me the job, but she has to give me the interview." She absolutely would not, so I came back the next day with a letter to the vice president. I called the Equal Employment Opportunity Commission (EEOC) and they said, "We don't cover you [discrimination complaints based on disability]." And I said, "Oh, no, this is not happening again."

> As a result of these things, I decided that the law
> had to change so I got involved [as a lobbyist].

Adrienne helped write the legislation that added disability to the other factors covered under the Human Rights
Law in New York State—age, sex, marital status, etc. The law
forbids discrimination in employment, private educational
institutions, housing, public accommodations, and credit on
the basis of any of these characteristics. She lobbied for the
bill until it passed in 1974. Adrienne feels she was invited to
apply for a job with the State Division in part because the
agency wanted a disability rights activist working inside and
not agitating about its failings from outside. Adrienne advises
would-be reformers that sometimes government agencies will
seek to hire them because they genuinely want their commitment to social change, but at other times, they will hire them
to keep them quiet. At the Division of Human Rights, she
handles all types of cases, but still takes a special interest in
disability-related issues.

To be a Human Rights Specialist—Adrienne's formal
title—you need a bachelors degree, community work experience, and a passing grade on a state examination. The first
position you are likely to hold in this field is Civil Rights Aide,
and from there you work your way up to Civil Rights Investigator. The salary for an Investigator starts at about $23,000
a year, increasing to $40,000.* The next step up is Supervisor
of Investigators, where duties include public speaking and
working with the community, as well as supervision of other

---

* The salary figures that appear throughout this book are rough estimates offered by the women being profiled. Salary levels vary over time and from one
geographic area to another.

staff. You could also use your training and experience in the civil rights field to do research or to teach. People at the very top in this field, who determine basic policies rather than work on specific cases, are appointed by the Governor and are likely to be highly successful lawyers.

Adrienne was born totally blind. Her parents moved from New York to New Jersey because New Jersey had a program to mainstream blind children. For kindergarten, Adrienne went to her local public school. From first to third grade, she went to another public school where she learned braille for part of the day with ten other children who were also blind. Braille is a method of reading and writing for blind people, where letters and words are formed by tiny upraised dots on the page so that they can be felt instead of seen. Adrienne hated the way the children in the braille program formed a separate group from the rest of the students. She wanted to be part of the whole school. By fourth grade, when she returned to her local school, Adrienne had learned to type her school work.

Although Adrienne's local high school did not strongly emphasize academics, she "survived" and "had a very good time in a lot of ways." She was active in the debating club and in the choir, worked on the yearbook and school newspaper, and also wrote a column for her town's newspaper. She had lots of friends, including a boyfriend who was a musician, owned a car, and adored her.

Every summer from age six to sixteen, Adrienne went to a camp for visually impaired children, sponsored by the New Jersey Commission for the Blind.

It was an interesting camp. I remember at some point—we were probably in junior high or around that age—saying, "Why is it if we can go to a public school, why aren't we going to [a regular] camp?

What's the logic of this? Is all this integration not
for real?" But it was a good camp in its way. It was
free; it went all summer. What it did was give kids
a chance to be together and compare notes about
how they were managing as the only blind kid in
their class. It was also valuable because kids of all
races, economic classes, and ethnic groups were
mixed together. For many of us who lived in all-
white suburbs, it was our first chance to know
blacks and Hispanics and anyone who did not have
our same background. I had experiences with kids
that were important for me and that were much
more broadening than the experiences of many of
my high school friends.

One of her camp counselors suggested that Adrienne
apply to Swarthmore College, which has very high academic
standards and was "not the kind of place my high school
would know about." She took the Scholastic Aptitude Test
(SAT), a standardized multiple choice exam that most colleges require of applicants. It tests high school seniors on their
math and reading skills. The testing service allowed her to use
braille for the tests, but then, without her knowledge, sent a
letter along with her test results to the several colleges to
which she had applied. The letter, called a "tip" letter, said,
"These tests were taken under nonstandard conditions," because of the braille. Adrienne believes she would have
strongly opposed such a letter had she known about it when
she took the test, and encourages other disabled students
facing a similar situation to protest. She states:

I believe that high school students and their
parents, teachers, and guidance counselors should
protest this "tip" letter, arguing that the so-called
"non-standard" conditions under which disabled

people take tests are the same "non-standard" conditions under which they will do their college and other professional work. For example, if they use braille, tapes, readers, other types of assistance, take breaks, or take more time than non-disabled people, they probably have been using these same methods to perform their work in the past and will continue using them in their future education and careers. Thus, the testing methods may not be "standard" for non-disabled people, but they are standard for the disabled test-taker and probably reflect how that person will do in performing work at the college or graduate level under these same conditions.

One college accepted Adrienne for admission, but administrators told her that they were afraid she would be unable to cross the street in front of the school. Swarthmore, however, readily admitted her with no reservations about her blindness. At Swarthmore, Adrienne took notes with a slate and stylus (a small, portable, quiet device by which the user writes braille on any type of paper; it is the equivalent of a pencil and paper), typed her papers, and used readers to help with assignments.

Adrienne has some strong feelings about how colleges should treat disabled students. She feels that the most important part of Swarthmore's—and any school's—policy on disabled students is that admissions be based on the same set of factors that is applied to non-disabled students, such as academic abilities, talents, and interests. Disability should *never* be used to screen out a student who meets the rest of the admissions criteria. After you get in, according to Adrienne, it's up to you to make the most of it. "It is not a matter of do they give you twenty-five special things once you're admitted."

After graduating from Swarthmore, Adrienne spent two years working at a variety of jobs and experiencing more than 100 instances of job discrimination—the episodes which led her to become active in disability rights. She states:

> Had I not had a history of political activism, in civil rights for blacks and in opposition to the Vietnam War, I might not have been so ready to fight for my rights as a person with a disability. I realized I would have to take the energy I had put into social change for other people's benefit and use it to benefit myself and other disabled people.

Adrienne then went on to earn a Master's degree in Social Work (MSW) at Columbia. At first, Columbia was reluctant to admit her because it did not believe that a blind person could do the community organizing work that would be part of her job. At the time, there was no federal or state civil rights law to protect Adrienne against these discriminatory attitudes. (Such laws were passed well after she graduated.) So she used her powers of persuasion and her strong conviction that she was competent to do the work to convince the school to allow her to proceed. In fact, she handled the work well.

After getting her Master's degree, Adrienne worked as a program analyst for the New York City Health Services Administration, looking at programs and deciding whether or not they were doing an effective job. In her spare time, she worked on changing the New York States Human Rights Law to include disability. Eventually, she left the Health Services Administration to take the job she holds now at the New York State Division of Human Rights.

Adrienne is now studying for a Ph.D. at Columbia University Teachers College, and is writing her dissertation on the way that people form their political beliefs. She's focusing on people's attitudes toward the Baby Jane Doe case. This case concerned a severely disabled infant whose parents refused to let her receive medical treatment. Some people support the parents' point of view, whereas others feel that the baby should have received treatment. Adrienne is attempting to determine what experiences and characteristics about a person influence how they feel about this case.

Adrienne also works as a psychotherapist part-time, helping people deal with emotional problems. In addition, she speaks, writes, and consults (advises people) on disability issues, and occasionally teaches a course on disabled people in American society. Someday, Adrienne would like to have a full-time job teaching social psychology (the branch of psychology that looks at how people interact with one another and how they feel about their experiences as a part of small or large groups, such as families, work, or school groups, racial or ethnic groups, etc.) and social policy in a department of social work within a university, To do this, she must have her Ph.D.

Adrienne says she balances her work life and social life "with difficulty." She hopes to marry and have children someday. Although she has had several serious relationships, she feels that her blindness makes it difficult to get relationships started.

> I am absolutely written off by people at parties, on the street. I'm looked past, ignored. Some of my relationships have started through music, some through politics, some through chance encounters. I've placed [personal] ads; I've joined dating services.

If friends introduce me to a man, they insist on telling him in advance that I'm blind, and they do it in a way that is an apology. I don't tell dating services that I'm blind. People are enraged. You think that employers are enraged about it [your disability] not being on your resume; well potential mates go bananas. If you put the blindness in, people won't respond, and if you don't put it in, people feel that you have deceived them.

Disability is neither at the center or the periphery of my life. It's just sort of there. I'm not saying blindness isn't an important fact about me or that it doesn't affect a lot of things, but it's not part of my self-definition. If it's part of the world's definition of me, that's the world's issue. I can't make it my issue.

Will blindness prohibit me from meeting someone? I hope not. At times I have been exceedingly despairing about the situation—but call me in a year.

Adrienne adds that while having a disability may make it more difficult to meet someone and start a relationship, it is not necessarily the reason why relationships do not work out. "Relationships may not work out because you and your partner find that you don't get along with each other, because you don't like each other's personalities, dress, work habits, friends, or families—the same reasons they do not work out for non-disabled people." She feels it is unfair—and inaccurate—to explain all of your romantic frustrations in terms of disability.

In her spare time, Adrienne likes riding a tandem bicycle (built for two riders), cooking, reading, and spending time with friends. She also sings.

I'm a reasonably trained musician and I work hard
at it. Being a singer who can't see is not so bad. You
can read and sing at the same time if you have the
music [that is, in braille].

When asked what advice she would give to teenage girls
with disabilities, Adrienne replies:

Don't start out your life with the questions, "How
is this going to prevent from doing X?" Or, "What
can I do because I have a disability?" That's not the
way to formulate that set of questions. The way to
formulate the question is "What do I want to do and
what do I have to do to get it?" If that means getting advice from disabled people, then by all means
go get it, but it may mean you want to do something
that you can't find any disabled person has ever
done, and that doesn't mean you shouldn't do it. It
just means that you have to figure out a way to
adapt what you want to do with your disability.
"What do you want? What interests you? What
friends do you want to make?" Not, "Is disability
going to be a problem with friends?" for example.
The answer is yes, it may be a problem. But they're
your friends and together you will figure it out. I
mean it's a problem that has a solution.
    Since there are a lot of disabled rights groups
and there are laws, know them, learn them, get in
contact. There is value to be gained from that kind
of affiliation. Don't overstate your disability and
don't ignore it, and don't think the only way to succeed is to act as if you don't have a disability, because in fact you *do*. And you'll need disabled
people somewhere in your life. Be assertive. Figure
out what you want and don't let people who say

you can't get there convince you that you can't do
it. Keep fighting, keep using your head, keep finding as many avenues toward where you want to go
as you can.

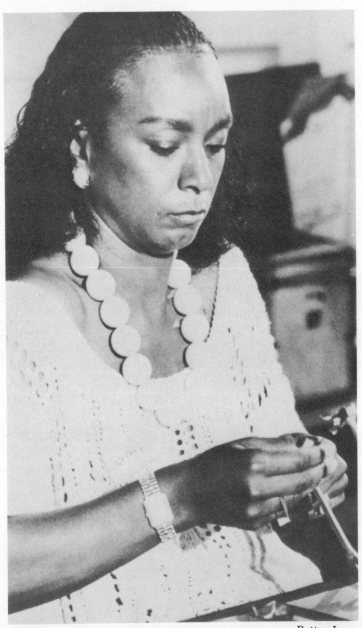

Bettye Lane

3

Barbara Cole-Appel

JEWELRY DESIGNER

Customer:	These emeralds are magnificent!
Barbara:	How are you going to use this ring? Will you wear it every day or do you want it to be the ultimate emerald ring for special occasions?
Customer:	I want to wear it on a day-to-day basis, but I want it to be the most important thing on my hand, to catch everyone's eye.

Barbara Cole-Appel, a jewelry designer, discusses a ring she is designing for a customer's birthday. Barbara has had her own jewelry business for several years on 47th Street in Manhattan, the heart of the International Diamond District. Paralyzed below the waist by a car accident when she was twenty-two, a year after she entered the jewelry business, Barbara does her work seated in a chair, surrounded by three work counters and a glass display case. Ninety-eight percent of her work is done by commission (a customer authorizes her to make a certain piece of jewelry within a certain price range). Barbara explains:

> I do basically what is called fine jewelry work.
> "Fine" means that it's done in precious metals:
> gold, specifically, and sterling silver. Occasionally
> I work with other semi-precious metals, such as
> brass and copper, but very rarely. And most of the
> materials used in combination with the gold are
> precious stones such as diamonds, sapphires,
> rubies, and emeralds.

Barbara usually designs a piece of jewelry exclusively for a client, and often along with the client. When a client comes in with a design that's not workable, she has to be a diplomat.

> I work with them on the basic idea whenever pos-
> sible. I try to improve the design concept so they
> visualize it differently. That's the delicate part of
> it. This happens very often because people visual-
> ize jewelry as being "this is what I want," but con-
> ceptually sometimes a setting or a style or a stone
> just doesn't work. You need a great deal of patience
> when you're in the design business. I make it a
> point never to "sell" anything to anyone, but just

to assist them in realizing what can be done or how something could be utilized. People trust you once they see you can help them and that's the key to selling.

After discussing the design with a customer, Barbara makes a model out of wax. This takes about two weeks. The model allows the client to see the product before its final state and before it has been cast into a precious metal. Using a model also gives Barbara a chance to make any necessary changes in the design by adding or removing wax. After the model has been created and refined, Barbara usually produces the actual piece within a week, depending on whether or not she does all the work herself. The prices of Barbara's jewelry range from hundreds to thousands of dollars a piece.

On a typical day, Barbara gets to work between 8:30 and 9:30 a.m.

The first thing I do is set up the display showcase, which means I take everything from the safe and put it on display. After that I organize for the day in terms of what work has priority. And then I proceed. All day long people come in and talk to me while I'm working. Sometimes it's difficult. Generally, when I really want to concentrate on something I'm doing, I will go in earlier so I'm less distracted. I don't want to be upstairs behind closed doors. That's why I have chosen to remain on the street level and highly visible, because I want them to see and feel my presence. When I am not in, I will leave a handwritten message in the showcase, and they can always call my answering service. People really like being able to touch base with you.

Barbara's accident happened when she was driving home from work one evening. She spent the next nine months in the hospital and a rehabilitative institute.

When I was told I was paralyzed, I had absolutely no idea what that really meant for me. What's paralyzed? It wasn't until I began to live a life outside the hospital and encounter the normal day-to-day process of coping with everything that I began to understand what effect my limitations had on me. Even now, in this fifteenth year of sitting in this wheelchair, my limitations change all the time. What perhaps I couldn't do in the first year that I sat in this wheelchair, I don't need to do now or I can do it in a very different way than I ever thought of doing it.

During her stay in the hospital, Barbara's parents were very supportive. Her father, who spent as much time as possible at the hospital (her mother was pregnant with her second child), convinced her that her accident didn't have to change her life.

My father literally lived in the hospital with me. He took a leave of absence from his work to spend time with me. He wanted me to understand that the accident did not have to change my attitude toward life. He made me aware that I was going through the very difficult stages. He said, "You have been altered in the sense that you're not going to be able to walk, but everything else that you were given is still here. You're still just as beautiful."

Like any person with a disability, Barbara had to deal with the way the outside world treated her. She says:

You must remember most people with any kind of disability are encouraged to take it easy, not to push themselves, not to expect too much of themselves. They have a reason not to do. This is basically what I kept hearing: "You cannot do this. You drive every day? You should not be driving." I really do not want to hear what I cannot do. It really took possession of me. I wanted to start my own company, but at that time I was afraid to venture out on my own.

Within a year of her accident, Barbara married the man to whom she had been engaged before the accident because her family and friends believed that this would be best for her. She felt they were saying, "No one else will love you. You are lucky someone loves you and wants to marry you." The marriage did not last. As a woman with a new disability, she was not yet ready to be with a partner. Barbara says:

I had to grow up and come into my own sense of self-worth and understanding. For the first seven years of being confined to a wheelchair, the key question in my life was "How am I able to take care of myself completely independently?" I wanted to know whether if I had to ask someone to do something for me, was it something I could not do for myself or something I could do for myself, but was making the choice that someone could also help me do it. It took me a total of ten years to know that I am completely independent and in charge of my own life. The next question was "How can I share my life with someone again?"

Barbara says she had to find out if men would still find her attractive and like her as much as before the accident. It was not an easy time for her.

> That was a pretty rough period for me because it meant that I had to go out and make myself available in a social environment. I would go to discos. I would get right out on the dance floor. I did not dance like anyone else, but who does? I did whatever I wanted to, moving my upper torso or whatever. And people were very receptive. I socialized with groups of people who were single and into dating, and I made it known that I was interested in meeting people. I had a ball.

Ten years after her accident, Barbara celebrated her independence.

> I flew to Hawaii and vacationed for two weeks, myself alone. The Islanders were curious because I was alone. One woman came over to me after a few days and said: "I do not really want to intrude, but I just want to tell you that you're the most magnificent person I've ever seen. We have watched you all over the island. The whole island is whispering how incredible you are." I felt I had been confined and now I was finally free. I also bought myself a very fine car and invested in a condo for myself. I felt I could make these important decisions that would permanently govern my life. I now knew what were right choices for me. I was saying "You are who you are and you are quite capable of having your business, your home, your car, and travelling wherever you want. You're a free person."

Barbara advises anyone interested in a career in jewelry design to start as an apprentice. Although Pratt Institute and the Fashion Institute of Technology have excellent jewelry programs, Barbara feels that working in the field is the best education. In a jewelry course, a person can learn the fundamentals—sawing, piercing, cutting, filing, setting stones. But, she says, it is necessary to know someone or "situate yourself in an employment position whereby you will be working with a jeweler or setter on an apprentice basis for five to ten years." Barbara looks for young students with talent, particularly female students, to work with her for short periods of time because she like to help them enter this highly competitive field. "It's a profession where no one is really willing to part with information because if you do you are inviting competition," she says.

Barbara graduated from Pratt Institute with a degree in interior design, a very difficult field for young people to enter. An interior designer helps people with the kinds of colors, furniture, and general decoration which would best suit their personalities and their houses. She or he advises the client, and then, with approval, buys the fabric, furniture, and paints, and supervises the actual work on the house. After working for nine months with an interior designer, she realized that she was unhappy because of her lack of independence. She would select the materials, while her supervisor or the department head would work directly with the client. In the future, however, Barbara would like to return to interior designing, this time working for herself, in addition to continuing to do jewelry design.

Barbara became involved in her jewelry work one year before her accident by investing in a jewelry company and then discovering she was extremely interested and talented in the field. Barbara says:

> I started working at the sales counter—it was a very
> big company. People would ask me questions
> about jewelry, so if I were going to answer, I had to
> learn the business. People began to say "You have
> good ideas, good taste, good judgment." Then came
> the accident.

When Barbara returned to work, at first on a part-time
basis, she realized that she wanted to be a jewelry designer.
Her mentor at the company, a woman who was a family friend
and a jewelry merchant, found it difficult to relinquish any
control of the business, so Barbara formed a partnership with
a woman who made wax models and was interested in getting more involved in jewelry work. Together they formed
CoJo Creations, Barbara's last name being Cole and her
partner's, Johnson. Barbara did the designing and her partner
would make the forms and models. After several years, they
dissolved their partnership, although occasionally the two
still work together. Now Barbara is, in her words, "a one-
woman show." She does all the designing, jewelry-making,
selling, and promoting.

Barbara likes the way her jewelry work makes her feel
about herself.

> It's very nice for someone to come along, look at
> what you conceived, developed, and made, and be
> willing to invest in it. That's a very rewarding feel-
> ing, that someone is willing to pay for your kind of
> ability.

Salaries for jewelry designers vary widely, usually rang-
ing from $250 to $1,500 a week. Owning your own business
gives you the potential to be more creative as well as earn
much more, or much less, depending on your business skill,
the amount of jewelry you produce, and the price you can ask

people to pay for it. The kind of people who do well in jewelry design have artistic ability and open personalities. Barbara says they "can relate and share with other people, and encourage them to be creative."

Four years ago, Barbara married a man whom she met when he came to her counter to have a piece of jewelry designed. She describes her husband, a highly successful stockbroker, as a "handsome, loving, sensitive man with a strong appreciation of art." They do a lot of travelling and both put their relationship ahead of their work lives. She has a three-year-old godchild whom she says is "an absolute delight," but she also knows that being a mother and not just a godmother would be "a major responsibility." Barbara is not sure if she wants her own children.

> I am living with a physical handicap and I wonder what kind of pressures it would place on the child as well as myself. I really like the freedom that my life offers me. I know that's really selfish, but it is my life. I like the freedom to be able to pick and choose.

At thirty-five, Barbara is happy with her life and feels she has come to terms with the paralysis caused by her car accident. She spoke of a friend who asked her if she would rather win a thirty million dollar lottery, be the most famous jewelry designer, or regain the use of her legs.

> I really had to think about it. I decided I would rather have the $30 million because losing the use of my legs has not inhibited me other than walking, as far as I'm concerned. Not being able to walk is something I have learned to live with. It's no longer something that I have to be able to do in order to feel complete. As far as being the ultimate

jewelry designer, to my customers I am. So let me have the money. I probably would spend a lot of time travelling. I would definitely organize some kind of training program for jewelers with aspirations. I'd have a major workshop in New York City.

When asked what advice she would give to teenage girls with disabilities, Barbara said,

If you feel there is something you want to pursue, you owe it to yourself to try. It isn't always necessary that you succeed. The point is that you tried. I think that is really important, because generally you accomplish, you learn something. There have been instances where I've approached things that I perhaps was not ready for, but I felt that I wanted to pursue, and sure enough I found I did get something out of it.

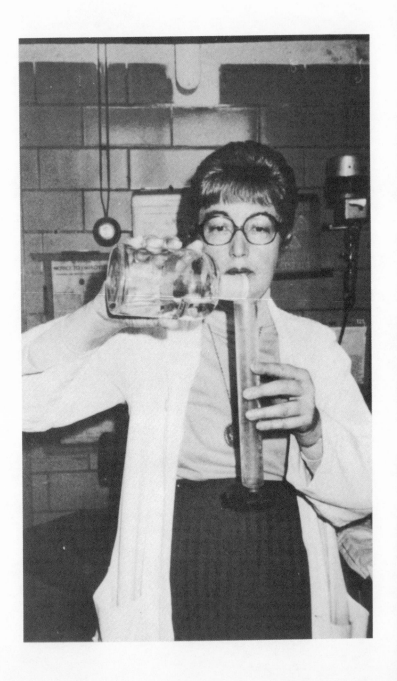

4

Nansie Sharpless

NEUROCHEMIST

"From the time I was very young I had an analytic mind. It was inherited from my father. The idea of not accepting things at face value without checking or experimenting first was part of my upbringing."

W hen Dr. Nansie Sharpless talks about her job, she uses complex words. Nansie is an Associate Professor of Psychiatry and Neurology, as well as the Lab Chief in Clinical Neuropsychopharmacolgy (the study of how drugs affect the mind and the brain of people with brain disease) at the Albert Einstein College of Medicine, in the Bronx, New York. She is also totally deaf as a result of meningitis (an infection of the membranes around the brain) which she contracted when she was fourteen years old.

Nansie has been at Albert Einstein since 1975. She works in her own laboratory, a small room crammed full of sample bottles and instruments she uses in her experiments. Psychiatry and neurology are branches of medicine concerned with the study, treatment, and prevention of disorders of the mind and the nervous system, respectively. Within the fields of psychiatry and neurology, there are many different areas of research. Nansie's particular area is called neurochemistry because she studies the chemicals that are manufactured by the nerve cells in the brain and released into the synapses, the tiny gaps between these nerve cells. ("Neuro" means nerves, and neurochemistry is the study of the chemical activity of the nervous system.)

The chemicals that Nansie specializes in, called neurotransmitters, carry messages from one neuron (nerve cell) to another. In normal amounts and combinations, these chemicals deliver messages that control a person's mood, temper, and body movement. They can, for instance, make a person feel energetic or calm. Sometimes, though, too many or too few neurotransmitters are released, which can cause depression, extreme tiredness, hyperactivity, restlessness, or impaired body movement (as in Parkinson's disease).

By measuring and analyzing the many different kinds of chemicals that travel between the brain cells, neurochemists like Nansie may be able to understand which chemicals affect which parts of the nervous system. This, in turn, may help them figure out how these chemicals and their effects can be controlled.

For instance, if a person has a tendency to get depressed easily, Nansie tries to find a certain chemical that causes this depression. Then she tries to figure out whether there is too much or too little of the chemical, or if there is problem in the way the nerve cells receive and respond to the chemical. The goal of her research is to come up with a way to balance the amount of chemicals in the nervous system, so that depression or hyperactivity can be controlled.

Dr. Sharpless did not become a neurochemist overnight—far from it! Nansie grew up at a time when very few women worked in the sciences, and even fewer stayed in school long enough to get Ph.D.s and M.D.s. She says:

> I grew up in the 1950s, and women didn't do things like that. They got married and had babies, and then they were involved in raising their kids and cooking and things like that...Though I *can* cook, I happen to be a neurochemist, too!

She says that her deafness was originally another inhibiting factor in her choice of careers.

> I thought that I wasn't able to do something like that...I had never heard of a deaf person with a doctoral degree. I always thought deaf people had to be sheltered, not ever meeting the public or anything like that—of course, they could never become teachers...

On the other hand, Nansie had many positive influences in her childhood that led her to choose science as a career. Her father, a biochemist ("bio" means a living thing, so her father studied the chemistry of plant and animal life), was her first role model. He used to bring home many of the things he worked with in his laboratory, and the family got involved in his research.

> My dad was originally experimenting in nutrition. Back at the time of the Second World War [in the early 1940s] he was experimenting with soybeans—ways to use them as food. He'd bring things home and we would have to try them out. And then there were also white laboratory rats—he wondered what they would taste like, and after other experiments with vitamins or foods they had to be thrown away anyway, so he brought some of them home. My mother made a dish for us and some of my dad's lab assistants once...

Nansie and her sister often went with their father to the Museum of Natural History when they were living near New York City, and the family frequently worked on puzzles or games involving problem-solving. One of the most important influences on her education was her family's religious background. They are Quakers—Christians who believe that there is "that of God" in every person and that there is no need for a formal creed or minister. They reject violence between humans, especially war, and they believe in the equality of all people. The Quakers' official name is the Society of Friends, which emphasizes the equality of each person within the group.

The Quakers strongly value education for both boys and girls, and Nansie thinks this helped her develop her strong interest in science and education in general. The stress in her family was on experimentation, not accepting traditional ways of looking at or doing things without at least questioning them closely.

Nansie, who is now fifty-five years old, spent much of her childhood in Detroit, Michigan. When she was thirteen and one-half, she moved to New City, New York. Soon after that, she contracted meningitis and became deaf. Although Nansie attended a special school for the deaf at first, she returned to her local high school in New City after her parents were advised that she would do better academically in a mainstream school. She started taking lip-reading lessons at the New York League for the Hard of Hearing, but since lip-reading takes many years to master, she was dependent on teachers writing extra notes on the board for her and on the notes of other students to keep up with the work. Nansie also spent a lot of time doing extra reading on the topics that her teachers had covered in class to make up for the discussions that she missed. By developing these strategies for learning, and working hard at them, she was able to do well.

When she got to Oberlin College, in Ohio, in 1950, Nansie continued to do extensive reading on her own as well as to borrow other students' notes to make up for what she could not hear in her classes. Following her childhood interest in the sciences, Nansie majored in zoology, the study of animal life, and by her senior year, she knew exactly what she wanted to do, which was to obtain a master's degree in medical technology and then go into medical research.

Nansie went through the master's program in medical technology with an "elite" group of women at Wayne State University in Detroit. These women were unusual because they were working toward advanced degrees at a time when many women did not even go to college. She got a job as a laboratory technologist at Henry Ford Hospital in Detroit, and from 1956 to 1967, she worked in two different departments. In one department, she worked on experiments involving chemicals from the adrenal gland that influenced hypertension; in the other, she did research on proteins found in the fluid surrounding the brain and spinal cord. Her work at this hospital introduced her to the field of neurochemistry, although she did not yet realize that this was the area she would specialize in.

After eleven years, however, Nansie found that she was bored. Her job did not allow her analytical mind enough to think about because she was always working on other people's research. Even though she still was not completely confident that she could do it, Nansie decided to go back to school and work toward a doctoral degree in biochemistry.

Nansie's decision was influenced by friends who had already followed the same career path.

> I was part of a group of women who had gone through the same program and had gotten Masters degrees, and then had gone back to school to get Ph.D.s or M.D.s—so that my friends were doing the same thing...I was a little bit behind them. Some of my closest friends worked for a little while as medical technologists and then went back to school. Just as they finished and got into jobs, I became confident that I could do the same thing. I wouldn't say that these women *encouraged* me to do it, but they stimulated me. They were all somewhat like role models—women who became professionals.

She started out slowly, working in the daytime and attending classes at night. She gained a lot of confidence during this initial period of studying part-time. "When I went back to school," she recalls, "I discovered that I could get good grades if I wanted to..." Eventually, she won several fellowships and was able to work toward her doctoral degree full-time.

In 1970, after four years of study and after completing her own research project, Nansie fulfilled all the requirements and got her Ph.D. In that year, the women's movement was also gaining strength and influence in the United States. More and more women were beginning to study the sciences and Nansie was in a position to help many younger women and serve as a role model. She was also fortunate to have had as an advisor and role model a woman who was working on the treatment of Parkinson's disease through the use of the experimental drug, L-dopa; this was a growing area of study. Under her advisor's influence, Nansie did her doctoral research on L-dopa and thus got involved in an area of neurochemistry with good career possibilities. After getting her Ph.D., Nansie spent four and one-half years in Rochester, Minnesota, where she did post-doctoral research on L-dopa in a laboratory at the Mayo Clinic. Then she came to Albert Einstein as an Assistant Professor.

She describes the typical career path in the academic world.

> The usual way to move up is to have post-doctoral training, and then get either a position as an instructor or assistant professor. This would depend on your teaching skills and your publications. Then ordinarily you stay as an assistant professor for about seven years. You are then evaluated for promotion to associate professor. This is the big hurdle, because you must have recommendations from people outside your institution—at least three. So it means that you have to establish a professional reputation away from your home institution. The promotion is based on your teaching skills, your service to your institution, the quality of your research work, and your publications.

To become a Full Professor, the next step up, you must establish a national reputation as a researcher and scientist, and you must publish many papers and studies in your specialized area.

Nansie works with graduate students at Albert Einstein, teaching them research methods and helping them with projects they must complete in order to get their degrees. She also conducts seminars (small discussion groups in which both students and professors present papers), and periodically gives talks to groups of students.

Nansie works with almost an equal number of female and male graduate students, but this does not mean that she thinks discrimination based on sex has disappeared from the sciences. It still is more difficult to be successful in the scientific fields if you are a woman. Nansie feels she has not always had all of the opportunities for advancement that she has been entitled to, given her abilities and background. But it has been hard to sort out which discrimination directed at her is based on the fact that she is a woman, and which is based on her disability. Despite some progress, it is still too often assumed that disabled people, like women, are incapable of mastering technical fields such as neurochemistry and other sciences. Nansie is continuously challenging this false assumption, not only for herself in her own career but also for other disabled people.

Nansie spends a great deal of her spare time encouraging young people who are deaf (and those with other disabilities, too) to look into the sciences as a possible career. She gives her time to organizations like the Alexander Graham Bell Association for the Deaf, the American Association for the Advancement of Science, and the Foundation for Science and the Handicapped, to provide young people with "living evidence" of success for deaf women in science. "I've given a

lot of talks oriented toward encouraging people who are disabled to enter science careers," she says.

Nansie believes that people with disabilities should
reach as high as they want to go, although they should do this
with a clear idea of the limitations their disability may im-
pose on them. "If science is you, then there is something in
every part of it that you can do."

Neurochemistry is an ideal career for Nansie. It taps her
intense curiosity and analytic mind. Her work in no way
depends on hearing, but rather on her mind's ability to
analyze what she sees in her experiments. Indeed, her
laboratory is organized to provide her with a visual way of
doing almost everything. For example, when timing her experiments, she uses a stopwatch rather than a timer with a
bell on it. She looks rather than listens to see if the water is
on or off, and watches the dials on instruments rather than
listening to them.

In her day-to-day work and home life, Nansie's deafness
is mostly an inconvenience. She has a telephone with two
receivers in her office—her secretary listens to each caller on
one receiver, transmitting an outline of what the caller says
to Nansie, who reads her lips. Then Nansie talks into the other
receiver. Nansie also has a TDD (telecommunication device
for the deaf) at work. A TDD looks like the keyboard on a
typewriter attached to a one-line TV screen. When the
telephone is hooked up to one, each person types rather than
speaks his or her part of the conversation. The words are sent
over the telephone wires and printed out on the other's screen,
where they can be easily read. For group meetings, Nansie
uses an oral interpreter (who sits across from her and mouths
the words of each speaker), since she may not have a good
enough view to lip-read for herself.

At home, Nansie has a closed-captioned television,
which means that spoken dialogue is printed at the bottom of

the screen and made visible with a special decoder. Her door-
bell works by flashing a light in each room of her apartment,
and her alarm clock is a timer which turns a light on at a certain time. In short, for Nansie, everything that you would
normally *listen* to is converted to something that can be *seen*.

Dr. Sharpless says that there are times when her disability causes discomfort and misconceptions among her
colleagues and her students.

> Sometimes it's difficult to get students to talk to
> me; some of them are a little bit nervous about in-
> itiating things. And so I have colleagues who have
> known me for a long time, who say to them "you
> have to go talk to Dr. Sharpless..." Once they get
> over this initial worry, we often get along just fine.
>
> It has taken a long time for people to realize that
> I might go to a meeting on my own and present a
> paper...or, people who don't know me don't real-
> ize that I drive. I still recall seventeen years ago,
> when the wife of our department chair said to me:
> "Oh, Dr. Sharpless, I think you're so wonder-
> ful...do you shop?" And I thought to myself, "How
> do you think I'm eating—my family sending CARE
> packages?!" There's lots of underestimation, or
> *non*-estimation, going on all the time. You have to
> establish a professional presence with people, col-
> leagues, who are worried about whether you can
> cross the street alone or not! We're not on the same
> level all the time. And sometimes they have the
> feeling that I'm brighter and more intelligent than
> I really am, too.

The best advice Dr. Sharpless can give to young women
with disabilities is to look all over for the thing you would
like to do.

As a young person with a disability, you should look at all careers and pick out the things you like to do best. It's important to enjoy what you do first. Then you should consider how your disability will fit into this. Any kind of career has something in it that a disabled person can do. But I don't think that you should ignore your disability or limitations. You should look for something very interesting to you, and also how it is able to accommodate your particular disability.

Author's Note: Sadly, Nansie Sharpless died of cancer in October 1987. Her friends, family, colleagues, and students miss her tremendously.

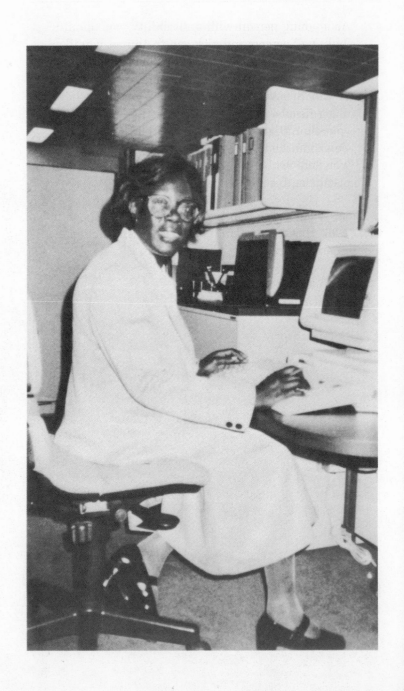

5

Linda O. Young

<u>SYSTEMS ANALYST</u>

User: The computer output is not in the format that our department needs. Can you help?

Linda: Come on over and let's talk about it. Let's see if we can change the program to meet your specifications.

Linda O. Young is a Systems Analyst for Metropolitan Life Insurance Company in New York, helping people at the company figure out ways to do their jobs more efficiently through the use of computers. She also has osteoarthritis, a condition that causes her hip joints to weaken, making walking and sitting difficult (she walks with a cane), and multiple sclerosis, a chronic disease of the central nervous system that causes Linda to feel quite tired much of the time. Linda explains, "Although I have had arthritis since childhood, it didn't necessarily prepare me for acquiring yet another disability—MS—as an adult. Living with two disabilities has been tough, but I have become even more determined to get my life together."

Linda has worked at Metropolitan Life since she graduated from college and moved to New York. Although she didn't start out in the company as a Systems Analyst, she moved in that direction because she felt it was an exciting, growing field.

Metropolitan Life is a large, multi-faceted company involved in developing and selling many different types of insurance policies that protect individuals and businesses against financial losses resulting from accidents, illnesses, death, fires, thefts, and other types of losses. To function effectively, the company must keep track of an enormous amount of information, such as the features of the various policies it sells and data on people who buy them. Computers have made this work a lot easier because they can rapidly store and analyze large quantities of information in many different ways. Of course, computers can only do these things with the help of people who tell them what to do. That's where systems analysts like Linda come in.

Systems Analysts at Metropolitan Life work in a variety of ways to help computerize the company. Sometimes they begin by meeting with members of a department to find out what types of tasks they do. For example, one department might be responsible for comparing the level of sales of different types of life insurance policies.

The analysts then design a system which will accomplish the task—in this case, to collect and compare the sales data of the various policies—through the use of computers. But their job doesn't stop there. Once they develop a system that is cost-efficient and has been approved by management, they teach members of the department how to use the new system, they "debug" or solve any problems which come up, and they improve the system over time so it keeps up with the progress of the company—for instance, expanding the system to include information about a new type of insurance policy.

Systems Analysts work closely with the people who use the computerized systems—called "users"—and may be on call in the evenings and on weekends as well as during working hours to provide assistance, since computers are often in use 24 hours a day. In the example presented above, the user needed the computer to print out the results of its data analysis—called the "output"—in a format that was different from what was currently available. Linda came to the rescue by figuring out a way to tell the computer—through a change in the "program" or instructions to the computer—to produce the output in a different format. "It's important to have good people skills as well as good technical and problem-solving skills," she says. "You sometimes have to calm people down while keeping calm yourself and you often have to deal with a lot of pressure. At the same time, it's thrilling to be able to solve a difficult problem…"

Although Linda has worked in New York for many years, she is not a native New Yorker. She and her three brothers and three sisters grew up in Pensacola, Florida. She describes herself as a "regular tomboy" until she turned eleven, when she began to have problems walking. At first, the doctors thought that placing pins in her hips would help her. But after two operations, when she was eleven and again when she was twelve, it was clear that the procedure was not doing the job, and she continued to have pain and difficulties in walking.

Linda describes her condition.

> Osteoarthritis is the deterioration of the joints. It could be any joint, such as your hip, knee, what have you, and it can affect you all over. There are times when my hands are not moving the way I want them to move—I used to have trouble screwing tops off jars, and things like that—but it has really zeroed in on my hips. The joints just deteriorated there.

After one of her early operations, Linda returned to school, continuing almost as if nothing had happened. The only difference was in the way she got to school.

> I can remember that, whereas everyone else in the neighborhood walked to school, my parents arranged for the school bus to pick me up, and I was taking the bus to school everyday. Later on, I remember riding to school with the teacher across the street.

"I guess I was popular," she says. "I had a lot of friends. I can remember being happy..." Did she feel "different" from the other kids? Yes and no.

> I was mainstreamed. I was never made to feel different from the kids and the people I grew up with. I knew that I *was* different, and I knew there were certain things that my friends could do that I could

not do. I knew that I had certain special privileges,
in that the bus picked me up and didn't pick up
anyone else. But I was never *made* to feel different
in a negative, rejecting way.

Even though her mother was a nurse, Linda says that she
never discussed her disability with her family when she was
young.

We never talked about it. Never. Even now, my
mother and I never talk about it. We talk about
what's going on now, but never about those days. I
think it was bad. I got special treatment from the
nurses when I was in the hospital, because my
mother worked there. But with all her training, she
never talked to me about it.

Her parents, she says, were not the type to talk about
anything "personal" with their children, so it wasn't just her
disability. On the other hand, Linda didn't press her parents
to talk about personal matters.

I didn't have a lot of curiosity—I find that interesting—and I don't know why. It's just like I can't
remember [much about her later childhood]. Now,
you don't say "boo" to me without me asking ten
million questions. For example, I have tremendous
curiosity about MS and read all I can about it. But
then I didn't have the curiosity. I knew that something was wrong...but I don't know, maybe in my
own way I went into a little shell—I didn't question. I think maybe part of it is that I took my cue
from my parents.

In addition to not wanting to go too deeply into personal things, her parents were very protective.

> I come from a somewhat strict Southern back-
> ground, so my parents were protective in general;
> but their protectiveness was more so with me. I
> learned in later years that my parents told my
> brothers and sisters that they had to look after me,
> that I couldn't do certain things.
>
> They just tended to let my brothers and sisters
> do more, and say to me that I couldn't do more or
> shouldn't do more. I think that's a part of Southern
> background, too. Instead of encouraging you to do
> and do and do if you have a handicap, you were
> not really supposed to do anything. That was just
> their way.

Linda always expressed interest in making her own living—she originally thought she might like to be a secretary or a teacher, or be in some position in the business world. Even though they were protective, her parents supported her desire to become independent.

> My mother—and I relate more to my mother be-
> cause almost everything was my mother—pushed
> like hell for me to go to college. I remember her
> saying that I should get some training so I would
> be able to support myself.

But her mother also thought that it would be essential for her to marry. That created problems between mother and daughter, particularly when Linda was younger.

> I think my mother was under the impression that
> no matter what, you should be married. I think a

lot of Southern parents feel that way. I think that
my mother felt that because I had a disability, I
should, more than my sisters, be married—I would
need someone to take care of me.

My mother used to be very upset that I was not
married. When I was in college, there was this guy
that I was dating, and he used to come home with
me. My mother loved him, and he told my parents
that he planned to marry me. We *had* planned to
get married, but things did not work out. And my
mother blamed me, and she told me that several
times. I think that—I graduated ahead of time, and
he was older and stayed behind—we just went in
different directions.

I had another chance, someone from my
hometown who lives here in New York asked me
to marry him—right before I went into the hospital
in 1971. And I said "no" because I felt there were
too many problems about myself and my physical
condition that I had to resolve *by myself* first.
Again, my mother was upset. I think now she's
come to terms with my reluctance to rush into marriage.

Linda attended a predominantly black college in
Florida, where she started as a secretarial studies major. "And
then I said, 'What am I doing? Can this really give me the kind
of future I want?' I decided to switch to Business Administration." Linda felt that this would give her more options than
secretarial training. The only accommodation Linda needed
while at college was a waiver of the physical education re-
quirement. Other than that, her college life was pretty much
the same as anyone else's. When she graduated, she had no
idea what she wanted to do with her degree.

Linda finally decided to work for the Metropolitan Life Insurance Company because she was eager to move to New York, a city that had always fascinated her. She also felt that such a large, diverse company could offer her many different career directions. Her first position there was as a correspondent in the Personal Life Insurance Department. Personal life insurance is one of many kinds of insurance sold at Metropolitan Life; it pays survivors, such as family members, a certain amount of money when the person who buys the life insurance policy dies. Linda worked with the company's district offices (local Metropolitan Life offices throughout the country that sell policies), helping them make additions or other changes in policies to reflect the individual needs of customers as well as changes and improvements in what the company was offering. Her job required lots of writing (most of her contact with district offices was through correspondence) as well as a strong knowledge of the insurance field. Since Linda had no prior experience, Metropolitan gave her extensive on-the-job training.

After several years in this position, Linda decided to move into the Personal Annuities Department. An annuity is a type of retirement insurance in which people put aside money when they are younger, and are then guaranteed a certain amount of money each year when they get older and retire. Linda's position within this department was called "Methods Analyst," which meant that she helped to solve problems to insure the efficient use of staff, materials, and equipment.

After working for a few years in annuities, Linda became interested in working with computers and applied for a position in the Electronics Department. She was hired as a Systems Analyst and was fascinated by her new job.

I began to move like hot cakes! I went to classes in programming for about nine weeks and my interest in computers kept growing and growing. The more I learned the more I wanted to learn. It was a tremendously exciting time.

Systems Analyst jobs like Linda's usually require a Bachelor's Degree in business, the sciences, or computers. Or you could qualify with specialized training in computer languages, start out as a computer programmer (someone who develops a set of specific instructions that tells the computer to perform certain tasks, and often works alongside the analyst) and then move up to a Systems Analyst position by learning on-the-job. Systems Analysts work in all types of settings from manufacturing companies to scientific plants to government agencies to banks to insurance companies. Although the specifics of the job vary and may require a particular type of expertise—for example, a chemical company may require a background in science, a bank, experience in finance—the overall goal is the same: to develop new and improved ways to computerize tasks within the company. As more kinds of businesses and agencies look to computers to assist them with their workload, the demand increases for Systems Analysts. The salary range for this job varies from $18,000 for entry level positions to $37,000 and up for a highly experienced person.

Linda says that computer-related work is a very good field for young women with disabilities.

It's a lucrative field, with many opportunities. Once you are trained in the basics, you can use your knowledge of computers in almost any line of work, and you can ask for a high salary, if you're good.

Linda chooses not to mention her disability on her resume, because she does not feel that it has anything to do with her job or her ability to do the work. Her disability has never been an issue among colleagues or supervisors, she says. When she needed a hip replacement operation last year, she was granted several months off for surgery and recovery, with no difficulties from her boss.

Linda feels that being a black worker in the predominantly white insurance business has been more of an issue for her than being disabled or being female. At times, she has faced stereotypical attitudes and prejudices. As she says, "Some people really underestimated me. They expected me to take long lunches and they did not think I was smart enough to take on the really interesting projects." At various points in her career, these prejudices made her doubt her own potential and her ability to make it in the insurance field. An important experience that helped her build her confidence and realize that she could make it was becoming the editor of a newsletter, *Intercom,* which was put out by Minority Interchange, a volunteer-run organization and support network for minority employees working in the insurance industry.

It was around the time of her recent hip replacement operation that Linda discovered that she had multiple sclerosis. She had been feeling tired and had greater difficulty than usual walking. These symptoms were not alleviated by the operation, as she had hoped. She went through an extensive series of tests and was ultimately given a diagnosis of MS. MS is a disease of the brain and spinal cord that involves a hardening of the tissues around certain nerve fibers, interfering with the brain's ability to control such functions as seeing, walking and talking. MS affects different people differently, and the same person can have different symptoms over time. Although Linda's main symptoms at present are extreme tiredness and the dragging of her right leg, she anticipates that at some point, her physical functioning may be more seriously limited and she may find it necessary to work on a part-time basis. She states,

> My plan now is to take several technical courses and learn as much as I possibly can about computers while I am feeling O.K. so that later on, should I need to work part-time, I will have my choice of jobs. Having a condition like MS has really made me give a lot more serious thought to my future and what I want and need to do for myself.

When she was younger, Linda had a tendency to shy away from social situations where her disability would be evident. One way her friends helped her out of this shyness was by gently forcing her to enter a room first instead of hiding in the rear of the group. More recently, Linda has not found it difficult to meet people, and she has learned to teach her friends just how much help—and how much protectiveness—she needs. Some of her friends don't seem to realize that she needs *some* help, and others tend to think she needs more help than she does.

Although she feels like a social person, Linda also enjoys solitude. "Sometimes I feel I'm a loner," she says. "I can stay alone at home for weeks and be perfectly content with my books and my home and myself."

Linda has been involved in a few relationships in recent years although she is not currently seeing anyone on a steady basis. She finds herself becoming more and more selective over time. "I really know what I'm worth and what I contribute to a relationship," she says now. "And I demand that a man recognize that in me and not mistreat me in any way."

In some ways, Linda wishes she were now involved with a man who could help her get through difficulties in her day-to-day life—and in more difficult times, like her long recuperation after the hip replacement last year. But she has serious doubts as to whether she will ever meet a man who can fully satisfy her needs, or with whom she could be totally compatible. She explains, "Especially with the uncertain course of multiple sclerosis, I am a big responsibility for myself, for Linda, and I could be a big responsibility for anyone else. But I'm not closing the door on the possibility."

Linda has some advice for young women with disabilities, and some of it is based on the mistakes she made when she was young.

> Don't do what I did. Don't take a back seat. Don't dwell on your disability, but don't run away from it, either. Take time to look at yourself. Don't let your disability hinder you. Don't use it as a crutch. Cope with it, make it comfortable for yourself. Whatever you do, don't let anyone put you down. Value yourself, and realize your worth, and realize you're a person too. You have a lot to offer, so offer it. Go for it!

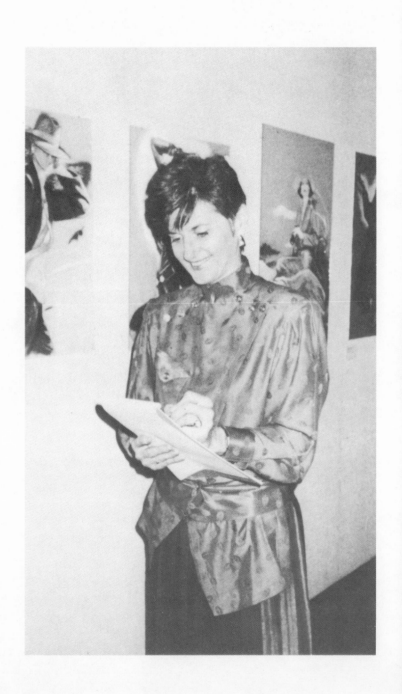

6

Dorothy Wainer

ADVERTISING EXECUTIVE

Scene: a carpeting manufacturer's office

Dorothy:	What is new about your product that you want to sell to consumers?
Manager:	We've developed a stronger fiber that makes the life on the carpet longer.
Dorothy:	What kinds of things come to mind when you visualize this fiber?
Manager:	Strong ropes, pyramids, strong vines...

Dorothy Wainer is Vice President and Management Supervisor of a New York City advertising firm. She has a partially paralyzed leg and hip as the result of a bout with polio when she was eleven. Dorothy loves her job, and she defends advertising against charges that it makes false claims about products.

> A lot of advertising goes on that is very productive and important. It provides a valuable service—an honest one. It's a question of the products you pick and how you advertise them. Advertising does get information to people.

But what exactly *is* advertising? It's difficult to explain because it is such a "non-specialized" field. But, to start off with, there are two sides to it, management and creative. The management side handles relations with clients—people, like the manager of the carpet manufacturer above, who have products that they want to sell. A person working on the management side of advertising, called an Account Manager, gathers detailed information about the client's product from meetings like the one presented above, and then works with staff in the creative department of the advertising firm to come up with an effective way to present the client's product to consumers. The resulting advertisement, through images and words, has to convince consumers to buy the product.

Dorothy graduated from Syracuse University, in upstate New York, with a bachelor's degree in advertising design. She had always been deeply interested in art, but could not see herself pursuing the fine arts, as opposed to commercial art, as a career.

> I thought of fine arts but knew I wasn't good enough to do it, and I wasn't driven to do it and become a

poor, starving artist for the sake of art. It just wasn't
in me to do it, and I knew that.

She came to New York because it is one of the centers of
advertising (along with San Francisco and Los Angeles) and
because it was close to her family on Long Island. But she had
no idea about how to find an advertising job, and no connec-
tions that might help her. She was, as she now recalls, "scared
out of my wits!" Finally, after a year of searching, she settled
for part-time work at a small advertising firm, as a
switchboard operator.

Determined to make it in advertising, Dorothy worked
for free at night in the art department of the same firm, learning the basics and showing the people in that department that
she could do the work. After about a year, she was rewarded
with a transfer to the art department. Working full-time,
Dorothy started at the bottom, doing "mechanicals" [pasting
and mounting type and illustrations according to a design
done by someone else; mechanicals are then sent to a printer
or engraver for reproduction]. Again, she volunteered her time
to do more complicated layouts and campaign concepts until
she got another promotion.

Working in a small ad agency gave Dorothy a chance to
learn many different sides of the business because in a small
office everyone does a bit of everything. For example, in addition to creating the advertisements for products, she was
able to make direct contact with clients, giving her a taste of
the management side of the business. In fact, she liked this
aspect of advertising so much that she decided to go back to
school to get an MBA (Master of Business Administration) degree, so that she could switch to management.

Dorothy got her MBA from New York University. She
entered NYU with no background in business, and without
the math skills that are very important in the field. After work-

ing a ten-hour day, she went to classes in the evening—for five years. She says it was like "torture!," and she almost gave up after the third year.

She received her MBA in 1974, and changed over to a management position permanently. She now has one of the highest positions of any woman in her company, and she oversees several different accounts, from an athletic shoe factory to a shipping company to a toy manufacturer. She says this is one of the most exciting things about advertising. "There's always something new—it's diversified. I have worked with dozens of different products."

These days, says Dorothy, people who want to break into the management side of advertising should specialize in the liberal arts in college rather than concentrating in business subjects. Agencies want future account executives to be "well-rounded." Both men and women who hope to end up in management often have to start at the bottom as secretaries, at salaries sometimes beginning at $12,000 to $16,000, depending on their education level. The salary can go as high as $100,000, however, if you are willing to work long and hard for many years.

If you prefer the creative side of the business, you should get a degree from a school of design, such as Parsons School of Design, the School of Visual Design, the Fashion Institute of Technology, or Pratt Institute, all in New York City, or the Rhode Island School of Design. Starting salaries at this end of the business are also low, although here, as on the management side, you can work your way up to a comfortable salary level after a few years. Starting salaries are $13,000 to $16,000, but if you are talented and innovative, you can make up to $200,000.

Polio (a viral disease of the nervous system which often results in muscle paralysis or weakness, now preventable through a vaccine) has made some things harder for Dorothy than they might be for other people, but she feels it has not been a major obstacle in her career or any other part of her life. She came down with the disease in the middle of sixth grade. She remembers:

> For some time, my parents and the doctor didn't know what it was. Until I couldn't walk and collapsed, they thought I had a cold. In those days there was nothing they could do about it. They took me to a hospital and just let it run its course. They gave me orange juice, and that was it. We just hung out until the fever went away, and then they gave us whirlpools and hot baths. Then they literally "stretched" us, because that's what they thought would help. My muscles tightened up incredibly. I couldn't move for weeks. And then they decided that the best way to stretch me was to sit me up. It was unbelievably painful. To me, it was what they would do to a prisoner of war in torture.
>
> At first I was paralyzed from top to bottom except for one arm and my head. After a month, little by little everything started to come back, and then I was left with what I have now, a paralyzed leg and hip.

Dorothy was out of school for most of that year, attending classes with other patients in a one-room schoolhouse at the hospital. But the kids at her public school did not forget her.

> I was very lucky. I had a very good support system. The class sent me presents and cards every week with my parents, and my parents came every Sunday. And there was this boy, called Tommy Ewing, who saw my picture and knew I was in the hospi-

tal. He decided that I would be his girlfriend when
I returned from the hospital. He didn't know I'd be
coming back with a lot of metal, crutches and
everything. But it didn't matter, he was in love...

When Dorothy returned home, she lived pretty much the
way she had before she got polio. She even continued to ride
horses, despite the doctor's reservations.

I was in love with horses as a kid, so I worked at a
pony track before I had polio. Afterwards, I used to
watch one of by best friends ride. She finally said,
"Why don't you ride?" I saw a girl with an am-
putated leg riding—she had a prosthesis [artificial
leg]—so I said if she can ride with one leg, I can
ride with one leg. I took off the brace—I was about
fifteen—and I learned to ride without anything.

Eventually Dorothy learned to walk without braces,
crutches, or cane. She walks with her knee locked, and sits
on her hip. Her disability makes her walk more carefully than
most people have to, and she says she falls more often than
her friends who use leg braces and crutches. But other than
that, she gets along without much trouble.

Dorothy says that her disability is not a major barrier in
the advertising business.

Advertising is a head business, not a foot business.
Disabilities don't have anything to do with your
head. Advertising has to do with how you think,
how you plan, how you orchestrate. All you have
to do is sit behind a desk and be creative.

On the other hand, being a woman in advertising does
mean having to deal with obstacles.

When I first got into the business, I had to overcome the fact that I was a woman. Because in those days—and this was a long time ago, it's not so true today—women were not accepted in managerial roles. All clients were men, and men would not accept working with a woman. That's what I had to overcome. And I had to gain enough self-confidence about the business to be able to tell them to go to hell. It took me a long time to do that.

About her promotion to Account Manager, Dorothy says:

I wouldn't have made it without having a male mentor [more experienced advisor] to sell for me. He would go with me [to meetings with clients]— for one client, we went for a year before I could go by myself. I would take notes, act like a secretary, until the client had enough confidence in me and believed that, though I was a woman, I could handle his account.

Her mentor was her first employer, and she realized later that he had not really done her any favors.

Because I worked so hard, he needed me in the agency...I became angry later on in my life when I learned that he had used me, because I never really got my due and I was underpaid. And I learned that I shouldn't have to apologize for being a woman, and I shouldn't have to be pre-sold. I recognized this *years* later.

Although Dorothy says that the discrimination against women is not nearly as strong today, there are still some restrictions. For instance, she could never manage an account for an automotive company, she says. As a Vice President, she is two levels from the top; above her there are Senior Vice Presidents and the top executive or Chief Executive Officer. "I could become a Senior Vice President, eventually—but never a top executive. And that [Senior Vice President] would take a long time, it would be hard to do." And though she is officially "second tier," she says:

> I'm really outside the second tier because I'm the only woman Vice President in management. I'm not part of the "good old boy" meetings. In fact, I'm not invited to all of them. They're very proud to say that I'm a woman Vice President; they use me when they need to.

But Dorothy also says that at times there are advantages to being a woman in advertising. Women tend to handle accounts that have to do with "women's products," and there are many of these. There are also a great many women clients now, which lessens the male domination over account management. On the creative side of the business, women with talent can advance to a fairly high level.

According to Dorothy, clients *are* sometimes uncomfortable about her disability.

> They notice something is wrong, but don't know how to handle it...I bring it up with clients, because I know people are curious and don't like to talk about it. Sometimes it comes up because people say, "Oh, did you hurt yourself?" A lot of people don't notice because I don't carry a lot of equipment with me.

But she often manages to turn her disability into an asset, providing her with a way to discuss with clients some strategies for getting their ideas across to consumers.

> Sometimes I bring it up because we talk about life experiences. We're talking about confrontations, learning situations, how to turn negatives into positives and problems into oppor- tunities...everybody's got their story about what they learned in life and what made them learn it.

The creative thinking Dorothy has used in advertising also helped her bring her adopted son, Mark, into her life. She decided, a few years ago, that she really wanted a child, but had not met any man she wanted to marry. Since adoption agencies have waiting lists of up to three years, Dorothy decided to find a baby to adopt on her own. She placed advertisements in newspapers and magazines, and hired a lawyer to make adoption arrangements. She finally located a young woman who had decided to give up her child. She had already broken up with the child's father before knowing she was pregnant, and felt she was too young and too poor to raise a baby herself. Thus, Dorothy became a mother. The biggest obstacle in Dorothy's search to adopt a child had been the fact that she is single; no one had a problem with her disability.

When Mark was a baby, Dorothy did everything she could to make carrying him easier.

> I've gotten every single device in terms of transportation. I have two kinds of strollers, a snug- gli carrier [a sort of a pouch strapped onto a person around the neck and back, in which a young child sits against a parent's chest, so that a parent can carry a child and still have his/her arms free], a sassy seat that straps the child in position on a

parent's hip, a backpack, and a cane—anything so
I don't lose my balance. I have fallen several times
with Mark—it's interesting how you protect the
baby. I ended up hurting myself, but he was never
hurt.

Mark, now a toddler, has brought much joy to Dorothy.
She arranges her schedule so that she can spend as much time
as possible with him.

In the mornings, I stay home late with Mark. It's a
very important time, the beginning of the day. So I
may do some of my work at home, and leave at
about 10:00, having started work at 9:00 while he's
around doing his thing, and he plays...They don't
ask me to go to early morning meetings unless it's
absolutely necessary. To compensate, I work
straight through lunch and as late as necessary.

Mark has been an influence in the balance between
Dorothy's personal and work lives. She says:

I don't work as hard anymore. I used to be a
workaholic, but I stopped. I discovered that it
wasn't healthy. I take time, I have new priorities. I
don't bring work home on weekends anymore.

Dorothy has always tried to keep her work and private
lives separated from each other, and has been fairly successful.

One way I did it was to spell my name differently
so that no on can reach me at home unless I want
them to. My business name is W-a-y-n-e-r, and my
private spelling is W-a-i-n-e-r.

Most of her social activities, while not directly related to her work, involve some project. She finds that working with people on projects provides her with a good way to get to know them. Good friendships and dating relationships sometimes develop as a result. For example, Dorothy is an active member and on the Board of Directors of Advertising Women of New York, an organization that enables women to network and support one another in what is still a man's world of advertising. Also, she recently met a man while horseback riding who had an idea for a program to prevent breast cancer in women. The man was a doctor and needed some help in making his project known to women in the New York area. Dorothy came up with a name—the Breast Health Program of New York—and a brochure that publicized the program. She also dated him.

In her advice to young women with disabilities, Dorothy says:

> Go for it. If you want something, there are very few people who are going to stop you. If you show signs of being a leader and want to take on responsibility, there's more than enough to do out there. There are not enough people who want to take on responsibility and follow through in this world.

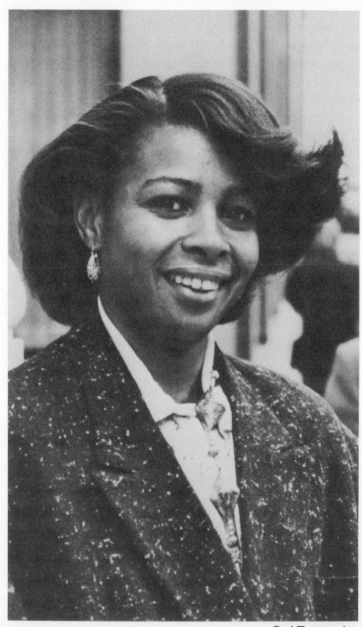

Geri Tommasino

7

Geri Strong

ACCOUNTANT

Geri:	But it's Tuesday! Tomorrow is payroll!
Junior Accountant:	I'm sorry. One of the day care reports was inaccurate and the computer kicked it out, so the City has given us no money to pay people tomorrow.
Geri:	Citibank will cover the $85,000 but can we get an emergency loan from the Executive Board?

Geri Strong, the Accounting Manager for the YWCA/YMCA Day Care Corporation, is in charge of payroll—recording employees' names and the money to which they're entitled, as well as making out their paychecks. She also handles every other financial aspect of the Corporation's eight centers every day. Geri has kidney insufficiency, which means that her kidneys work at less than their full capacity. This makes it necessary for her to spend a good part of the day in a hospital three times a week, undergoing a treatment called dialysis.

Geri says that problems like the payroll crisis described above occur much more often than she would like because:

> We get our money from the City [New York City] and if you've ever dealt with the City, you know they operate on a schedule akin to the man in the moon. The City takes its time in doing things. They think nothing of giving us our payroll check right on payday rather than a few days before like they should, and they don't care if it takes three days for their check to clear.

During a typical day, in addition to working with the payroll, Geri pays bills for each of the eight centers, for anything from milk to electricity; gets money from the City, from fees paid by parents with children enrolled in the centers, and from other sources, and makes sure they are deposited correctly; and literally accounts for every penny that comes in and goes out of YWCA/YMCA Day Care. For her work, Geri is paid $22,000 a year.

Although her job is very stressful, Geri likes it because "there's a beginning and an end in accounting, unlike some jobs that go on and on." She also likes the independence she feels on the job, and the fact that she is an accountant for a non-profit day care corporation is important. She says:

I'm not too interested in the profit end of accounting. It doesn't make me feel good to see the numbers accumulate on the page. I like it the other way around, when I can spend it all and bring it down to zero. Oddly enough, it is important because in day care they give us a set budget—$200,000 to $700,000, depending on the size of the center—and this is the budget for the year. There is no such thing as carrying over what you have left to the next year, nor is there any such thing as getting more money if you have a budget overrun. There are guidelines; they don't tell us what color of crayon to buy, but they do tell us we have to buy crayons and paint.

Most of the money to run the Day Care Corporation comes from New York City agencies like the Agency for Child Development, because most of the 1,500 children who come to the centers each day are from families with very little money to pay day care fees.

When she was nineteen, Geri was walking to the store when a car sideswiped her, ran over her foot, and threw her backward onto a cinder block near a construction site. Her foot was not broken; in fact, she felt nothing initially except her bruises from the fall, but she ended up spending nineteen weeks in the hospital. A week after the accident, Geri says, she developed what first appeared to be a cold.

The doctor thinks that I had some kind of break in the skin and an infection. That's what really did it: trauma to the area and an infection on top of it. The accident just set off a chain reaction. I had a 104 degree fever, which is pretty high for a nineteen-year-old. My kidneys failed during that fever. I was at home and I turned grey. I also had a funny odor, like urine. They rushed me to the hospital and I was there for what seemed like forever. They tested my kidneys and put me on dialysis. There was some kidney regeneration afterwards. Now it's insufficiency, not failure. They [the kidneys] function at about 42 percent of their capacity.

The kidneys are organs that remove bodily waste from the blood. They take byproducts from the food we eat that are not useful to the body and break them down so that our bodies can get rid of them. If the kidneys are not working properly, this waste builds up, causing illness and, eventually, death. In order to prevent this from happening in her body, Geri is "hooked up" to a dialysis machine, which helps her kidneys filter out the wastes in her blood.

Geri has a renal shunt, a sort of socket, implanted in her leg, which is where the machine hooks up to her. She has a dialysis session early on Sunday morning, one on a weekday evening, and another on a weekday afternoon, for which she leaves work early. Each session lasts from four to six hours, and though not painful, can be uncomfortable at times. There is a buzzing, a vibration from the machine that she can always feel.

The buildup of waste makes Geri feel "dizzy to the point of fuzzy" by the time she goes to the hospital for a dialysis session. On Thursdays, the day she has her afternoon session, she often "can't think straight" by the time she leaves work.

Those are the days I leave accounting alone and do a lot of the other paper work, like writing letters. Sometimes on the way to work, I'll look out of the train and say, "that stop looks familiar; I think I was supposed to get off there." And I'll sit there for two stops before I realize I was supposed to get off. That doesn't happen too often, but it does happen. The accumulation of wastes—it takes your energy, your attention span.

On the other hand, after dialysis Geri is often "wired."

My children and my man are used to it. Two o'clock in the morning and I'm still talking. After dialysis I go home, but before, when I used to go to the day care center after dialysis, I had to go get a letter from the doctor stating that this was common behavior, that I wasn't on cocaine.

During a typical dialysis session, Geri sleeps, reads, talks, or does needlepoint. Sometimes the partitions separating dialysis patients are removed and a psychologist leads a group therapy session—"when they have us all stuck there and we can't go anywhere," Geri says. She has made some very close friends among the other patients and the nursing staff at her dialysis unit. In a way, the hours of each session are protected time when she can be with friends.

Geri is surprised when people classify kidney insufficiency as a disability because she doesn't really think of it that way. She says it is only disabling "when I'm hooked up to the machine and I'm not mobile." But it does limit her ability to travel. She can only go to places where she can make arrangements to have dialysis, and she must make plans for this at least two weeks in advance. When her grandfather died, for instance, she could not go to his funeral because she couldn't make these arrangements in time.

When it comes to co-workers and friends, Geri says she would prefer not to talk about her dialysis at all. She says that she used to want to talk because *she* needed to—it helped her get used to the changes her disability made in her life. All in all, however, Geri has decided that telling co-workers causes more discomfort for them than it's worth, especially since her dialysis only rarely affects her daily relations with them. Sometimes though, because her condition is invisible, her co-workers become confused by her sluggish or "wired" behavior before or after dialysis. Then she will offer the needed explanation about her disability.

Geri's job in accounting is only one of several kinds of positions you can hold in the field. For example, you can start as a bookkeeper (a person who keeps a record of all the money which comes into and goes out of a business); ten bookkeepers currently work under Geri's supervision. To get this job you need a high school diploma with some additional bookkeeping courses. To be an accountant, you usually need a B.A. (four years of college). An accountant analyzes financial information, does financial statements, prepares payrolls, and fills out tax forms. Accounting Managers need a B.A. and experience in the field. The salary for an accountant at a non-profit agency ranges from $13,000 to $30,000; the range is higher in for-profit corporations. Bookkeepers earn less money and have less responsibility. A Certified Public Accountant (CPA), an accountant with a B.A. degree who has passed an extensive state-wide examination, can make a considerably higher salary.

While Geri knows she could earn more money in the corporate world, and has even been offered higher paying jobs, she prefers to stay at the Y because she enjoys and believes in the work she does there. In fact, Geri has no interest in becoming a CPA. She says:

> I'd rather balance the money that is there rather than try to amass it into a fortune. I guess I'm not that ruthless. I'm not interested in profit. I'm not interested in finding tax loopholes for people. I'd rather spend it the way we do than try to accumulate it, parlay it here, shuffle it around there, and

get it into zero coupon bonds [a bond that you buy at a discount, but that you don't get interest on until you cash it in, after about five years—so you make a profit from investing, but it takes longer than with other kinds of bonds].

Geri graduated from Brooklyn College with a degree in biology, though she did take accounting courses there. She then earned a nursing degree and was a Registered Nurse for almost six years at Brooklyn Jewish Hospital. Eventually Geri came to the conclusion that nursing did not fit in with her personality—she "cared too much, probably because I had been in and out of hospitals so much." She says that she got very involved with her patients and found it hard not to try to help them emotionally as well as physically. Most health care professionals, she says, learn how to treat their patients as "patients" instead of people, and this keeps them going through years of working with illness and death. She "burned out," and decided to change jobs.

Geri chose accounting because it was so far removed from health care. She would not be dealing directly with people, but rather with numbers, so there was not a potential for the kind of "burn out" she experienced in nursing. She left nursing and returned to school, this time to get a graduate degree in accounting from New York University.

Geri got her accounting job when she stopped by the Coney Island Day Care Center to visit her friend. According to Geri:

I just went to say hello and she was nuts with the payroll. She said, "You wouldn't know how to do payroll, would you?" And I said, "As a matter of fact, I do." I ended up working there for about two years, and then I was transferred to the Roberta Bright Day Care Center [also in Brooklyn]. Because of problems with fiscal management, the City gave the centers to the Y [asked the Y to take control of their accounting]. When the position of Accounting Manager became available, they offered it to me. And here I am.

Accountants need to like to work alone and pay attention to detail. Geri says:

If they [accountants] need people, they're in the wrong business. To be an accountant, you need to be good in math and be able to concentrate. If you don't like details and you don't like investigation, it's not the field for you. You could be literally looking for two pennies a day, and you have to want to find those pennies. You can't feel that it's *only* two pennies—accounting is very precise. When I find the two cents out of a million dollars, there is a thrill involved, a thrill of accomplishment.

Although she really does enjoy accounting, Geri's love of the health care profession is still strong. Her ideal job would be as an Accounting Manager at a large hospital. That way, she could be involved with health care but not in such an emotionally draining way.

Geri sees accounting as a good field for people with disabilities. It doesn't require a lot of physical strength or manual dexterity, just good concentration, skill in working with numbers, and the ability to get to and from the job.

Geri was raised with her brother and sister by an aunt and uncle, who adopted her. She says her adopted parents pushed their children. They were "all into [the idea that] black people have to achieve." They stressed independence, managing money, and education with all of their children. Her parents also influenced her love for medicine and her decision to become a nurse. Her brother, similarly influenced by them, became a doctor. After her accident and kidney failure, Geri's parents were extremely supportive.

> My family was the reason I didn't stop school alltogether. I was very angry with the world. Why was I singled out? My family were the ones who said, "You're stronger than that. What makes you think the world owes you a living?" Had it been left up to me, I would have gone on welfare and stayed there. I hate to say that, but it's true.

Joseph, Geri's husband, was also a support for her after the accident. The two had been friends throughout their childhood.

> He was the friend who came most often, who brought me the McDonald's hamburger when I got tired of hospital food. Now he makes sure I take my medication and constantly questions me if I went to the doctor. He's very involved.

Joseph and Geri have three daughters, ages ten, thirteen, and sixteen. Doctors warned her against having children, but she felt that her body could take the stress.

> They absolutely did not want me to get pregnant. But I didn't have a minute's trouble. They watched me very carefully—I had a doctor's appointment two times a week from the beginning. The length of dialysis was longer and they increased it by a day. Nothing happened, not even a Caesarean [a method of delivery where the doctor opens up the mother's abdomen and removes the baby, often be-

cause normal delivery would endanger the
mother's life].

Aside from her work and home activities, Geri does
needlepoint, rides an exercise bike to keep fit, and walks a lot.
She has twice walked thirty miles for the March of Dimes
Walkathon. Geri has also taught handicrafts at her church in
her old neighborhood.

When asked what advice she would give to teenage girls
with disabilities, Geri stressed the importance of accepting
and realizing the potential advantages of your disability.

You have to come to a point where it's O.K., what
happened to you, and not allow it to beat you up.
I've found that my disability in a funny kind of way
was a blessing. You have to look at the good in it.
A lot of people walk around every day and they
don't have pain; they're not appreciative of that.
Suddenly when they get a headache, it's a big
traumatic thing. People who have disabilities often
look at the world differently. We share that attitude
of living day to day. I don't have pain today, and
that is something to be thankful for. Also, if you
have a disability, it's important to recognize how
much you really can do. Don't let people tell you
that you can't do something if *you* think you can.

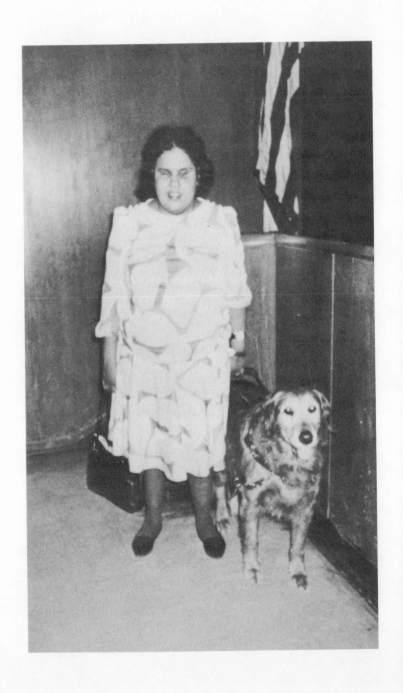

8

Alice Crespo

COURT INTERPRETER

A witness testifies in Spanish in the Criminal Division of the
New York State Supreme Court. Alice Crespo translates.

Witness:	Me robaron dos veces y me dieron plata por que ellos querían que nos mudaranos.
Alice:	I was robbed twice and given money because they wanted us to move.

The witness is cross-examined.

	Did you have any heat or hot water?
Alice:	Tenía usted califacción o agua caliente?
Witness:	No.
Alice:	No.

Alice Crespo, the first Spanish-English interpreter for the New York State Supreme Court who is blind, stands with her guide dog, Xenta, next to the witness. As the witness testifies in a landlord conspiracy case, in which the landlord has been accused of harassing and bribing tenants to force them to leave, Alice translates quickly and precisely, in a quiet yet authoritative voice. All eyes in the courtroom focus on her. As Alice says, "I'm always on stage."

For six to seven hours a day, Alice translates for Spanish-speaking defendants and witnesses in cases involving murder, robbery, homicide, and other felonies punishable by more than one year in jail. She also contacts the relatives of defendants to explain to them in Spanish the outcome of the court procedures, including prison sentences.

Alice loves her work. She describes it as a great opportunity to meet lots of different people and to learn about many different lifestyles and ways of thinking. But it can also be pretty demanding.

> People don't always use proper language. You can't fix it up a bit. You must translate exactly. It helps knowing street Spanish [the expressions and shorthand words people use in day-to-day life, which are often different than the formal language]. Like they don't always know the proper medical terminology, so they use their own terms. They just whip it out and you have to whip it out that way. And you have to work very fast. The good thing is I don't have to look at everybody's faces.
>
> You're not supposed to interpret body language. If witnesses shake their head, you're not really supposed to interpret because that's not the

spoken word. The only thing you are supposed to
interpret is the spoken word.

Alice explains that to become a court Spanish interpreter, you need a high school diploma and a passing grade
on both a written and an oral test. The oral test involves translating from English to Spanish in front of a group of people in
a mock or "pretend" trial. The interpreter needs to know both
street Spanish and traditional Spanish. Alice adds that to be
a good interpreter, it helps to be outgoing and comfortable
with lots of different types of people. It's hard to be on center
stage in the courtroom if you are very shy or embarrassed. But
you can learn by doing, and you often become more comfortable the longer you work. Annual salaries for court
interpreters in New York range from $20,000 to $28,000.

Alice decided to become a court interpreter at the sug-
gestion of a vocational counselor. She graduated with a
B.A. from Hunter College in New York in 1978, knowing she
wanted a career but uncertain about what type of work she
wanted to do. She had majored in sociology in college and
had originally wanted to become a rehabilitation counselor,
but then decided she did not want to obtain the additional
education the job required. Alice went to the International
Center for the Disabled for job advice, and her counselor there
encouraged her to consider court interpreting because she was
fluent in both English and Spanish. Although Alice had never
known anyone who had become a court interpreter and had
never before thought about this as a possibility, the idea ap-
pealed to her. She passed the interpreter's test and her name
was added to the list of those eligible for court interpreting.

Once ready for work, Alice was quickly and painfully
confronted with prejudice against people with disabilities
when she was told on a job interview that "court interpreting
is too difficult for a blind person." The employer claimed that

she would have to do a lot of maneuvering around the court building, and that without sight she would never be able to manage. Outraged, Alice decided to complain to the Equal Employment Opportunity Office of the New York State Supreme Court, which handles all types of discrimination cases. The staff there advised her and her potential employer that she would have a strong discrimination case if she were not hired. So the court reluctantly agreed to hire her.

Alice explains.

The court had been afraid that one of the defendants might act up or hit me, or that I might otherwise get hurt on the job. There was also the fear that my dog might bite someone. I myself doubt it. I think the defendant would probably bite the dog sooner.

Because Alice had to threaten a lawsuit in order to get her job, her employer was not that willing to help her learn her way around the building or assist her to adjust to her new surroundings in other ways. She herself found it difficult to ask for the help she needed. She states:

Having braille indicators on the elevators would have made my life easier, but I did not ask for them because I felt I shouldn't make any special demands. Now, eight years later, I feel a lot more comfortable asking for what I need, but I feel silly demanding changes in the elevator at this point, when I have been using them as they are for so long. I guess asking for help is not yet as easy for me as I would like it to be. But it is an issue that all of us as disabled people need to keep struggling with—to make sure we get what we need.

Once hired, Alice also discovered that defense attorneys were uncomfortable with her blindness. They feared that her limitations might hurt their clients. However, Alice was able to educate these lawyers about her competence by the very act of working with them.

One particular lawyer said, "I don't want this interpreter because she can't see my facial expressions. Also, if I have to run up to the pens [the room in which defendants are kept when they are not in the courtroom], it will take her longer to get up there. I don't think she will be able to interpret so well." The judge denied his application [for another interpreter]. After that, he worked with me on three more cases, and now he thinks the world of me.

Despite the negative attitudes Alice initially faced, she is extremely pleased with her job. She feels that this field offers excellent opportunities for people with disabilities.

It is a job that almost any disabled person can do. If you are in a wheelchair you could do it because you just use your voice. If you are blind, you would have no problem. It is not a job that involves lifting or moving that much. You need to move from place to place, but even if you were in a wheelchair, you could use a motorized chair. Courthouses are fairly accessible.

After eight years as an interpreter, Alice is considering advancement to a higher position, such as Interpreter Supervisor, which would involve supervising the work of several interpreters, or Court Clerk, where her duties would include monitoring all of the aspects of the courtroom procedures, in-

stead of just translating for Spanish-speaking witnesses and
their families. Because advancement to these positions
depends mainly on scores on standardized tests rather than
on more subjective factors, such as personal interviews, she
is confident that prejudice against her disability will now be
less of a barrier to her career.

One of several children born to her Puerto Rican parents,
Alice grew up and still lives in the Williamsburg section of
Brooklyn, New York. Because she was a premature baby and
was placed in an incubator where she received too much
oxygen, Alice has been totally blind since birth. Her parents
had no prior experience with disability and were under-
standably unprepared for a child who was blind. They did not
know what types of assistance and services she might need
and how much to expect from her. Right from kindergarten,
they tried to mainstream her into the local schools. The
experience, as Alice now recalls it, was a difficult one.

> I don't think it is so great to be mainstreamed in the
> early grades. You are not always accepted by the
> seeing kids and you don't have any kids you can
> relate to. It can make you feel like an outsider. I
> think at the early ages I would have rather gone to
> a school for the blind because it would have been
> easier: the games, the gym would have been struc-
> tured to meet the needs of people who don't see.
> When you are older, say seventh grade, and you're
> more able to handle it, then you should
> mainstream. This way you could get half of each
> world. I think that combination might work better.

Although her parents expected her to attend regular
public school with non-disabled children, they had different
life expectations for her compared to her non-disabled peers
and siblings. Alice remembers:

My father and mother didn't expect much from
me. They didn't expect me to go to school and get
a job or get married and have children. They pretty much thought I would stay at home, where they
would support me and then the government would
support me. But I always wanted to do things
myself and refused to accept the idea of being taken
care of by my family or the government. I simply
told my family that I was going to college and that
I was going to get a job. They didn't much like the
idea but they had no choice.

"My parents came from Puerto Rico," Alice says, ex-
plaining their attitudes in terms of their culture. "There,
women stay home and raise babies. If you have a disability,
it is assumed that you can't or won't have babies, but you stay
home anyhow, being taken care of by your family."

Some of Alice's high school teachers and counselors also
had limited expectations for her. At times she would get dis-
couraged and think of leaving school because she felt that she
wasn't "the brightest student in the world." Counselors even
told her it was all right to quit. It was largely through the en-
couragement of her friends who were themselves disabled as
well as her own sense of commitment to herself that she was
able to finish. She says that "It is a terrible temptation to listen to people who think they know more than you, but the
reality was in this case that we were wiser than they were."

At Hunter College, Alice was able to get the school to
provide her with some of the equipment and assistance she
needed to do her reading, write papers, and adjust to campus
life. She persuaded Hunter to purchase a braille machine so
she could work on papers in the library, and she used readers,
who read to her in person or on tape, as well as the reading
service, Recordings for the Blind, to assist her with her

work. However, she faced many barriers on campus. She notes that money for readers was never enough to cover all expenses, and that professors often didn't specify assigned readings until the first day of class, which made it difficult for Alice to get the texts recorded in advance.

She also discovered that too often accessibility was defined for people in wheelchairs or with other mobility impairments, disregarding the needs of students like herself with other types of disabilities. "Administrators think that if they build a ramp into the building, all the problems of the disabled are solved."

After graduating from Hunter, Alice started using a guide dog instead of a cane. According to her, it was "like having a car when you are used to riding the subway." The dog enables Alice to find things more easily and to walk faster because she doesn't have to worry about obstructions.

Even with her dog and the various devices she uses to assist her in her daily life, Alice notes that she has limitations connected to her disability. She wishes that the world and disabled people themselves would find the acknowledgment of limitations and difficulties acceptable. She says:

> We don't balance the scale enough to make people feel it is O.K. to have certain limitations. You have to be either super-good or super-bad; there is no middle ground. It can be exhausting. Even today, if I am having trouble crossing at an intersection, I hear people on the street say "Oh, my Aunt Sylvia could cross no matter what happened. Her dog was marvelous. That dog never made a mistake." People cannot accept it can be difficult.

In addition to her work, Alice has been involved in Disabled in Action, an activist group that focuses on pushing for legislation to protect the rights of disabled people, and is responsible for providing accessible buses in New York City. She is also a founder of Independent Recreation for the Disabled, a group that arranges trips and social activities for people with disabilities. She formed this group in part out of her desire to have more social activities and opportunities for herself. As a woman with a disability living in New York City, she has found it difficult to find ways to meet people for friendships and particularly for romantic involvements. Alice finds it easier to relate to disabled rather than non-disabled people because of the shared experience around disability, but because of all the accessibility problems, there are not enough places to meet disabled individuals.

Although Alice is not currently involved in a romantic relationship, she hopes to get married some day. But while recognizing that other women who are blind do choose to become mothers, she is less clear about having children.

> I don't think I want children. I'd feel guilty. It is sort of not fair to them. My kids might want something that I can't give them and then I'd feel bad. But I don't say never [about having children] because in this life you can never say never.

Finally, Alice has this advice for younger disabled women.

> It is very important for disabled people not to limit themselves, but they need to look realistically at what they can and can't do. If they are picking a career where the disability does interfere, it is okay to say maybe it isn't suitable. To look at limitations realistically is as important as figuring out things you can and want to do. Disabled people need to sit down, preferably with other disabled people, and discuss the real pros and cons to every job or

whatever they want to do. And they shouldn't limit
themselves by choices other people make. They
should not be intimidated by agencies. The same
people who are always giving advice are not always
around when you need them. You have to be a person who can make a decision to suit you, that can
say "this is what *I* want to do." Disabled people
need to have more role models, not just "able-
bodied" people trying to make decisions they know
nothing about.

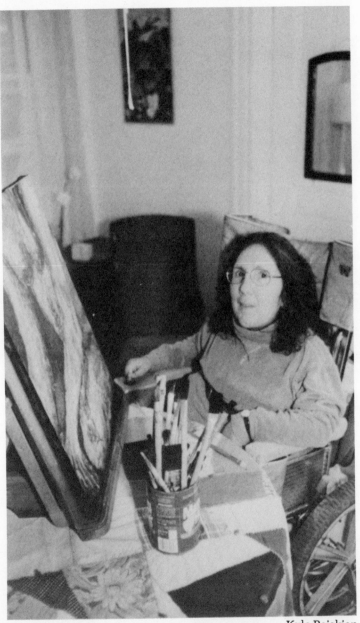

Kyle Bajakian

9

Connie Panzarino

ART THERAPIST

Johnny:	I'm making a mess for mommy.
Connie:	Yes. What do you want to do now?
Johnny:	Clean it up. And make another mess for mommy.

Connie Panzarino, an art therapist, has had Werdig-Hoffman's disease—a kind of partial paralysis—since birth. She works patiently and sensitively with Johnny, a four-year-old with cerebral palsy who has poor neurological control. In this session, Johnny, who had previously been fastidiously clean, made a big, yellowish-green mess with his paints and then asked if he could clean it up. He repeated the process several times. Connie discovered in the course of her work with him that Johnny did not have bladder or bowel control, and was upset that he was still in diapers while other kids his age could use the toilet. Connie explained to him that she has several friends with disabilities who also wear diapers. Johnny was amazed. She told him that sometimes her friends don't like wearing diapers, and that sometimes she didn't like to use her wheelchair, but that it is O.K. to use diapers or a wheelchair. He can still do all kinds of things and have fun.

Art therapy, according to Connie, is "wonderful, powerful, and fun." It involves using the media of art—pencils, pens, paints, clay, and crafts—to help people express their conscious and unconscious feelings and needs. She describes art therapy as "like when you dream and your unconscious [the part of your mind that you are not aware of] works out a lot of things. It's somewhere between that and being totally conscious and verbal about it [your feelings]."

Art therapy can be helpful to adults as well as children, she says,

> because most of us have problems: it's like surgery without the pain. You can get in there and work with the child in somebody without having them become childlike. What you go for is for someone to transform painful things that happened, the anger, fear, or whatever, into something much more tangible—using paint, clay, or crayons.

Art therapy is also useful in counseling couples. Connie will ask the partners in a couple what each hopes for as an outcome in their relationship, and each makes a drawing of it. Connie describes one session.

> In the woman's drawing, her ideal of what she wanted in the marriage was she was going out of the door with a suitcase on a trip. In his picture she was serving him a romantic dinner. They had a lot to work on. He was shocked and so was she. If they had to verbalize that to each other, it could never have happened, because you can't verbalize simultaneously.

In an initial art therapy session, Connie usually talks to clients about their previous art experiences, asks what they expect from art therapy, and suggests art materials for them to use in the session based on their answers to these questions. After clients finish a drawing or painting, Connie asks them to talk about it. Her goal is help them to find solutions to problems they are facing and to recognize their own strengths. For example, she says:

> If someone draws a duck being devoured by a lion, I will empathize with the duck, and I will also ask, "How do you think the lion feels?" I'll try to help the person feel both parts. I'll ask, "Is there anything that poor duck can do to help himself? Is there anybody else to help him?" I try to elicit a response.

Connie says that an art therapist can learn a lot about people through their art work. Things like lines, color, boundaries, and the size of a work can reveal much about a person's emotions. When Connie was struggling with issues of feeling separate from her family, for instance, she had a hard time coloring to the boundary line of an object in her drawings. Once she felt more separate and independent, she no longer had this difficulty. She is quick to say, however, that there are no "set answers. You can't say this always means that. You can't say a round house always means something because the person may have grown up in the islands where everyone has round houses. There's no set way of looking at a specific problem." In any case, Connie always praises and supports whatever drawings are made.

Connie often does art work along with a client, to show support and to further discussions. She describes each session as "an art work."

Connie was born with amyotonia congenita (or Werdig-Hoffman's disease). She has quadripareses, which is partial motor control of her arms and legs, and has 24-hour attendant service to assist her. She uses an electric wheelchair which she operates with the same finger she uses to paint and draw. Her head is supported by a headrest. Connie's spine is seriously curved and she has a speech impediment. She says:

> I'm not supposed to be alive. I'm the oldest person so far that my doctors know of with this disease. [She is thirty-nine years old.] It's very rare. Most children with Werdig-Hoffman's disease die before they are five. I finally asked, what do people with my disease die of? The doctor said, "They choke to death." I said, "Great. So *now* you tell me." Now I blend ninety percent of my food. If I go to a restaurant, I bring my blender.

In her work, Connie uses a table easel that tilts, and long sticks with pens, pencils, and brushes attached. These devices allow her a wider span of movement. She used to be able to hold brushes and pencils in her hand, but now she

puts them in her mouth. An attendant who follows her instructions to the last detail works with her in therapy sessions.

About attendants, Connie says:

> My attendant is an extension of my body. It takes
> a very emotionally as well as spiritually strong per-
> son to understand that and not resent it. If I don't
> direct the person, then I'm dependent on the per-
> son. Then I'm not autonomous and ultimately it's
> harder on the attendant. I make it very clear that
> I'm not making decisions for *them*, only for *myself*.

Until she was twenty-five, Connie's mother was her attendant. Connie was not able to get funding for a professional
attendant until she left home. Now she typically has three or
four attendants to cover 48- or 72-hour shifts. She says that
young disabled people often have a fantasy that they will grow
up and find the perfect attendant to take care of them for the
rest of their lives. This is not likely to happen, she warns, and
it wouldn't necessarily be a good thing anyway, because you
would become overly dependent on your attendant.

Currently, there are no licensing requirements for art
therapists; anyone can claim to be one. But this is changing.
More and more employers require that an art therapist be
registered with the American Art Therapy Association. The
AATA, in turn, requires a master's degree in art therapy and
100 hours of paid experience with a supervisor, or a certain
amount of course work and seven years' work in the field.

To get a master's degree in art therapy, you must take
courses in psychology, child development, psychological
testing and evaluation, drawing, painting, sculpture, and art
therapy. The mix of courses varies from college to college.
Some schools put more emphasis on art, while others are
more concerned with psychology. An art therapist needs to

be an artist in her own right, continuing her art even when she has a therapy practice, so that she won't become dependent on clients to express her artistic feelings. One of the most important qualifications, Connie says, is liking yourself.

> You have to like yourself or at least want to. That is a requirement for any therapist. If you don't like yourself, you will wind up working out too much of your own stuff with the patient. Because it is an unconscious process, if you are afraid of what's inside yourself, you won't be able to trust yourself to respond freely.

An art therapist can earn as much as $30,000 a year or more, combining work with community service agencies and private clients with the sale of her own art work. However, it is a fairly new field, with few agency jobs at the moment. Connie hopes this situation will change. She says that art therapists are working toward gaining society's recognition of the importance of their work. For instance, she says:

> Art therapists are trying to study the art of sexually abused children compared to the art work of other children, because the type of art work that those [abused] children do, other children don't do and don't know how to do. If we can prove this, then these children will never have to testify in court that they were abused. If their art was there, that could be admissible proof.

Connie's early education was at home. When she reached seventh grade, she was allowed to attend school for only half the day because there was no one to help her with the bathroom. Adjusting to school was hard for her.

At home I was used to being on my own, going at
my own pace. I was used to learning everything a
lot faster. I was bored a lot in school. My grades
were not that good the first year. I got C's. I was
talking in class—I mean, I had always talked in my
class. And then I was cheating, although *I* wasn't
really cheating. I was helping other students. I
didn't understand the competition, except to com-
pete with myself.

Once she got used to school, Connie started feeling pres-
sure to excel because she was the only disabled kid there.
"They wanted to see if disabled kids could do well in school.
If I screwed up, that was it."

Connie's younger sister also has Werdig-Hoffman's disease because it is hereditary, but a less severe case. Connie
describes growing up with her sister.

It was like having a twin, struggling with similar
issues around disability, but because I was twelve
years older, it was also like being her other mother,
giving support and advice. We both had to do
without getting our needs met quickly because my
mother was caretaking both of us. As a result, there
were enormous pressures on my parents, like
double work to take care of us, double doctor bills,
double guilt and frustration.

The doctors told Connie's mother that if she followed
their instructions perfectly, Connie would be fine by age ten.
This, of course, was not true. Connie also believed she would
be able-bodied when she grew up, because she had never seen
a disabled adult—she thought all adults were able-bodied. By
the time she was a teenager, she realized that her disability
was not going to disappear. On top of this, she had many

friends with muscular dystrophy and other disabilities who died when they were teenagers. She sometimes found herself wondering whether she might die too, since she was not going to be "cured." Connie describes these teen years as a difficult time of adjustment, and sometimes she had to battle against depression.

As a young child with a disability, Connie was often given art work to do to keep her occupied. She enjoyed art but never took it seriously. Until she was fifteen, she thought she might like to be a doctor, but decided she couldn't take laboratory science because she didn't know the lab tables could be lowered to wheelchair level. She explains, "No one was there to tell me about adaptations in those days." When she went to college at Hofstra University on Long Island, she majored in English and thought she would become a writer—even though at that time she hated to write. She says that writing was her mother's idea. "My mother felt writing was a realistic expectation because it was something I could do 'alone in my room.'"

Eventually, Connie discovered how much she liked art, especially watercolor painting and sketching. A career in art therapy was suggested to her by a vocational rehabilitation counselor. After reading some books about the field, Connie enrolled in the art therapy program at New York University, where she received an M.A.

Connie now works at the Boston Self-Help Center, which is a peer-counseling and advocacy agency for disabled people run by disabled people. She works part-time as the Executive Director, which means she "runs the agency, gets funding, trains and supervises counselors, speaks to able-bodied people about disability rights, and helps other disabled people feel good about themselves." She has also started an art therapy service there. Connie owns a van in which her attendant drives her to and from work.

On the issue of whether or not she includes her disability on her resume, Connie says:

> Of course. It's part of who I am. I don't want to be discriminated against. I'd rather they know it. I'm so blatant with it that they can't be sneaky and throw my resume in the garbage. My disability is an asset. I can see five clients who are disabled in the same time that a non-disabled therapist can see one because I don't have to figure out stuff about what it means to be disabled. I'm very vulnerable. I've been through a lot. I am open with my vulnerability and I am a strong role model. People see me as having done so much with very little, and I think it empowers them to do a lot with what they have.

Colleagues initially expect less of Connie but change their minds after a few weeks. She is always very direct. In a first meeting, when people try to shake her hand and find that she can't move it, she says, "'I can't shake your hand, but you can touch me if you like.' And I smile."

Connie's intimate relationships are now with women. She was involved with a man for several years, but realized that she was particularly attracted to men who had more female qualities. She became a lesbian, which means that she prefers to have a woman as an emotional and sexual partner. She says:

> I find defining relationships between two women to be very exciting because there are no set roles. I am not into roles. The bonding between two women is different than that between a man and a women. In addition to being partners, we are also like sisters and we can share everything.

Connie has been seeing a woman for about two years and is very happy in the relationship. Although her partner also has a disability, Connie explains:

> I have no preference between disabled and non-disabled partners. I wind up with disabled partners a lot because we share a reality. But some non-disabled partners can understand and offer that kind of sharing too.

Outside of work, Connie likes to cook, raise cats, write poetry, and garden. She has written an autobiography. She also holds workshops to help people become more sensitized toward disability, lesbianism, and other women's issues.

When asked what advice she has to give to teenage girls with disabilities, Connie replies:

> Get to know your body and find out what you can do and feel and what you want. Realize that you can be a sexual being. People tell you it is in your attitude and I do believe it because I'm much more disabled now but I also feel much more sexual. I know I am attractive and I know I can give and receive pleasure. Maybe my definition of sexuality is different too. I used to worry about what I could or could not do. Now if I can't do something, I just think of other things that I can do instead.

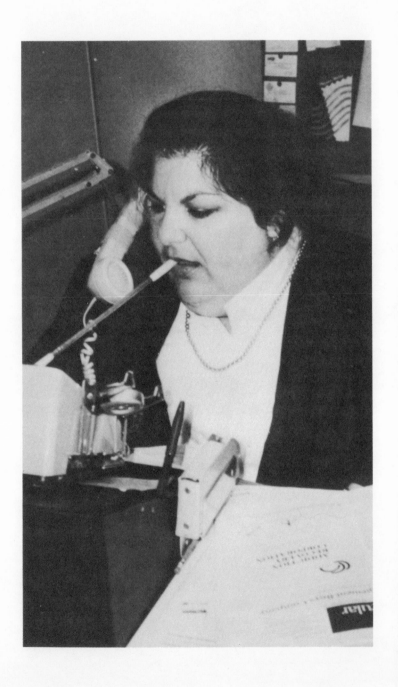

10

Carol Ann Roberson

VOCATIONAL REHABILITATION SUPERVISOR

Carol Ann: What schooling have you had?

Client: No school. They let me go only when it rained. You see, I work on a farm and picked cotton and...

Carol Ann Roberson, a supervisor of rehabilitation counseling at the Rusk Institute for Rehabilitation Medicine, which is part of the New York University Medical School, questions a southern black man, trying to find out about his background and what kind of work he likes to do. He is aphasic, which means he has difficulty speaking. At his second interview, he brought Carol Ann a piece of cotton to illustrate what he picked at his job. Carol Ann got him a job in a restaurant kitchen where he began washing lettuce, eventually working his way up to making pies. Then he became a hotel dishwasher. Now he is a bellhop at a New York City hotel, making about $350 a week.

Carol Ann, who is quadriplegic as a result of polio and uses a motorized wheelchair, provides job counseling to people with a range of disabilities. As a first step, she encourages her clients to fantasize about the type of work they might like to do. For example, she asks them

> to write down the kinds of things that they like to do. Then we pull out the qualities from these things that they find enjoyable. For instance, you discover that the person enjoys doing things alone, or maybe he or she prefers to be with lots of people. Then you make a sheet of the pros and cons of fifteen or so jobs that the client has heard about from family and friends and thinks he or she might like. You go through the list and ask, "What do you think you would like about these jobs and what do you think you would hate." And then you pull out the qualities from that and as you go along you begin to find that you have some issues to look at in terms of what kind of work is the person really interested in.

Carol Ann counsels both recently disabled people and those who have had disabilities from birth. For the last two and one-half years, she has also worked with cancer patients who are undergoing rehabilitation. She helps them deal with the reaction of others to their cancer when they return to work after operations, chemotherapy, or radiation treatments. In addition to her direct work with clients, Carol Ann supervises six other rehabilitation counselors. She meets with them weekly to review their work with clients, brainstorm problems, strengthen their counseling skills, and ensure that they meet reporting and other agency requirements.

Before she was hired for this job, Carol Ann graduated from Hunter College, and then earned a master's degree in social work in a two-year program at New York University. Although she was never trained as a rehabilitation counselor, she gained her certification in the field by passing a written examination developed and administered by the National Commission on Rehabilitation Counselor Certification. The more typical route is for a person to obtain a master's degree in rehabilitation counseling, which is also a two-year program, and then to take the certification exam, although not all jobs require certification in order to practice. The beginning salary for a rehabilitation counselor is $15,000 to $18,000. A supervisor can earn as much as $35,000 to $40,000.

Carol Ann got polio when she was five years old. The disease, also called infantile paralysis, damages nerve cells in the spinal cord. Until a vaccine was developed by Dr. Jonas Salk in the 1950s, polio epidemics were common. Carol Ann's illness left her arms and legs paralyzed.

There were a number of people on my block in Brooklyn who had gotten polio. This was right before Salk [the vaccine] came out and in fact there was a major epidemic in the Midwest. One of the

reasons that they believe my disability is as severe
as it is, is because there were no ambulances with
respirators [devices to help keep a patient breath-
ing] to take me to the Sister Kenny facility [a special hospital for polio patients located in New
Jersey]. They just let me stay at City Hospital. All
the ambulances with respirators had gone out west
to take care of the epidemic out there.

The oldest of four children in an Italian family, Carol
Ann grew up on Manhattan's Lower East Side. Once she became disabled, her fear was always that her parents would
move to some inaccessible new place in the suburbs.

At one point—I was about eleven—my parents
were thinking about buying a house. I can remember praying and wishing and doing all sorts of
things so they would never buy it because the
house was way out in Queens somewhere. All I
could think was, "I am going to be stuck on this little block in Queens with a tree, and I'll never be
able to do anything." Because I was close to the Village [Greenwich Village, a Manhattan neighbor-
hood], close to my friends, and uptown, I could go
and do whatever I wanted to, once I got my
motorized wheelchair when I was ten.

Carol Ann played with several close friends in her
neighborhood. For the most part, they adapted to her limitations, often in very creative ways. According to Carol Ann:

When we played jump rope, they would tie one end
of the rope to my chair rather than have someone
else turn it, so that I really participated. Or if we
played a game like skelzey [where you go from box

to box on a chalk board you make up on the
ground], someone would shoot my bottle cap when
it was my turn.

Carol Ann describes her parents as extremely
overprotective. They were reluctant to let her go out of the
house by herself or even with her friends for fear that she
would fall out of her wheelchair or be hurt in other ways.
However, Carol was quite adventuresome and social; she
loved to be out exploring the world with her friends. So she
had to figure out ways to work around her parents' fears. Carol
says she really appreciated what one girlfriend did. She
"crossed the street with my wheelchair 150 times when the
street had been freshly cemented to prove that she could cross
with me—through the wheelchair track marks—so my mom
would let me go to the movies with a group of kids." Often
Carol found herself "doing things first and telling my mother
later" in order to do the things she wanted to do. Eventually,
her parents became less fearful.

In the 1950s, when Carol began school, mainstreaming
was unheard of. Disabled kids didn't go to school with non-
disabled kids. So Carol Ann was bussed away from her
neighborhood to an elementary school with a class for disabled children.

I was bussed every day. I lived the closest to the
school, but they took the kids who lived furthest
away home first so I was one of the last ones to be
dropped off. That meant that I travelled around. If
I got out of school at two o'clock, I would get home
at five o'clock. It was horrible.

Carol also spent part of her elementary school years on
home instruction, which meant that a teacher came to her

house once or twice a week to provide lessons in all the different subjects.

At home, Carol had fewer hours of instruction than she would have received had she attended school, and no opportunity to learn with other children. If bussing was difficult, so was being required to stay at home.

Carol's parents were concerned that she was not receiving as good an education as her non-disabled friends. So they joined forces with parents of other disabled children to push the Board of Education to provide more and better schools for children with disabilities. In high school, Carol Ann was again bussed, but she was mainstreamed into the school, except for homeroom. The school had an elevator and was basically accessible. Carol Ann took whatever courses she wanted. Usually she took her own notes with a pencil in her mouth. Or she remembered the materials and wrote it down after the class. Occasionally, she would bring carbon paper and ask someone to take notes for her. Unfortunately, Carol Ann could not participate in extracurricular activities because she had to leave immediately after school on the bus. In the summer, however, she went to camp with other young people with disabilities. This was a good experience because "there was a real feeling of participating with other people, and not being different." She also got involved in crafts and singing.

After high school, Carol Ann attended Manhattan Community College and then entered Hunter College. She says she attend Manhattan Community College because she couldn't convince any other school to take her.

> The way that I originally got in was I wrote to then-Senator Keating and said I really wanted to go to school and the Office of Vocational Rehabilitation (OVR) would not provide me with transportation.

My feeling was either they pay for me now for the
next four years, or they could pay for me for the rest
of my life [with benefits] because that was what
was going to happen. It was a brand new school,
and I graduated with the first class after two years.

Then Hunter College accepted her, but not without
reservations. The administration at Hunter did not want to
give her any "special accommodations."

Hunter originally would not take me. Then they
said that if I ever asked anyone to help me go to the
bathroom, or do anything, they would expel me
from school. I was ushered into the dean's office
and told this. It was so devastating. Each time I
remember it I get goose bumps, it was so horrible.
I mean, it's scary to go to a school in the beginning,
to think you're going to meet people and worry
about whether you are going to be as good as they
are, and then to be told you better not want to go to
the bathroom!

While she was still at Manhattan Community College,
some of Carol's friends applied for a work-study program
(combining a part-time job with classes) and persuaded her to
apply along with them. Carol told them, "You've got to be
crazy. They're never going to hire me to do anything." But
they persisted, telling her she should at least give the counselor in charge of the program "a chance to say no."

Mr. Chase [the counselor at the school] really
looked and said to me: "If you can find a work
placement near where you live, we'll sponsor you
there." And so I went around and he called around
and someone had a contact with the Educational

Alliance, a tremendous old settlement house, three blocks from my house. And that's how I got my job as a lounge aide there. It was just answering phones, watching that no one stole the balls at the pool table, and that the radio was not too loud. This job eventually led to more responsible positions, and was a big factor in my decision to go into social work. Then, when I was in social work school, they said they couldn't find a field work placement [an internship] for me in my second year. That's when I suggested the Educational Alliance because I was still working there. You're not supposed to work while you're in social work school, but I had gotten a taste of the good life and I wasn't going to give that up.

Carol Ann met her husband Carl at the Educational Alliance while he was working with a youth program. They started off as friends and their relationship kept growing.

Carl and Carol Ann have now been married for fifteen years, and they have two daughters, Nicole and Giovanna, ages thirteen and eleven. Family life hasn't always been easy. Carl is black and Carol Ann is white. At first, Carol Ann's parents found it hard to accept her husband. They were concerned about the racial differences. Also, because of the severity of her disability, her parents had never expected her to get married. While they thought she would have a career, they could not imagine her living independently from them. They didn't believe that Carl or any husband would be willing or able to provide her with all the physical assistance that she needed. Carol acknowledges that she had similar fears at first.

How much could I ask this man to do for me? I needed so much help. On the other hand, I recog-

nized that everyone tends to overlook what I can
give. Disabled people are never seen as being able
to give; they're only seen as being able to get.

And both she and her parents had some initial worries
about her having children.

When my kids were younger, I can remember always being afraid. If something happened to Carl,
someone would possibly take my kids away from
me because the expectation might be that I couldn't
do it alone.

When Carol announced she was pregnant with her
second child, her mother's response was, "Are you crazy?!
Why would you do such a thing?" Carol Ann's mother was
afraid she would never be able to manage with two children.
Carol Ann's response was to get angry at her mother. She felt
that she and Carl should be entitled to make the same
decisions about the number of children they wanted as any
other couple.

In fact, they figured out a way to manage which has become increasingly popular today. They decided that Carl
would quit his job and become a househusband, staying home
with the children full-time, while Carol Ann continued to
work and support the family. They divided tasks within the
home. For example, Carol Ann was the disciplinarian and the
more organized one.

In raising her children, Carol Ann found alternative
ways to parent.

With my kids I learned to read upside down. I
couldn't hold the book so they could sit on my lap
and read with me. They could sit in front of me and
hold the book, facing them—so I learned to read

upside down and I can do it pretty well. It's not a
skill I'm going to use all the time, but it certainly is
a skill that helped in terms of doing a functional
thing with my children.

Time and experience put to rest any fears Carol Ann had
about being a parent. People too often concentrate only on the
physical aspects of childrearing, Carol Ann learned she had
a lot more to offer her children.

One of the therapists at work was saying to me,
"Your kids are so terrific. You really did a good job.
They are beautiful and I don't just mean physically. They're beautiful people. And I think that's partially because you work at those other kinds of
things that sometimes people leave out because
they are so into the physical."

Carol Ann often wonders how people see her and her
husband.

I think people have questions when they see us
together. I'd love to be in their minds. They think,
"What is he doing with her, and what does he get
from being with her? Is he a saint?" Carl *is* a special person, but not because he's done this sup-
posedly humanitarian thing of marrying me, a
disabled woman. It has more to do with who he is
as a person and how easily he can get past the ex-
terior of anyone. I've seen him in the elevator talk
to people who no one else has talked to in years.
That's the kind of person he is.
  There are men out there who come on to every
woman, but when they get to me, it is a totally different relationship. While on the one hand, a come-

on is not exactly what I want, on the other, I wonder how they see me. I am not the ideal of physical beauty, at least not the one that is in vogue. They probably think that I cannot give anything. They have a limited view of what giving and a loving relationship are all about.

When asked what advice she would give to teenage girls with disabilities, Carol Ann says:

Don't be afraid to explore and try. If it doesn't work, it doesn't work—but O.K., so you tried. It's just like anybody else. Things are not always going to go the way you want them to go, and that's not necessarily because you have a disability. That's because that's the way life is; it's tough sometimes. Things don't always work out. If you take a chance, it might not work out, but it *could*. And it wouldn't work out if you didn't take the chance.

Author's Note: Since this chapter was written, Carol Ann Roberson has moved to a new position as the Director of the Mayor's Office for the Handicapped in New York City. This office, which has a staff of forty people, serves as the link between the disabled community and city government. Carol Ann oversees new legislation, new ideas, and a range of services and activities of benefit to people with disabilities.

OTHER BOOKS BY AND ABOUT WOMEN WITH DISABILITIES

- Browne, Susan E., Conners, Debra, and Sterne, Nanci. *With the Power of Each Breath: A Disabled Women's Anthology*. San Francisco: Cleiss Press, 1985. This collection of personal stories, essays, and poems is a journey into the lives of fifty-four women with disabilities, who describe their experiences surviving in an inaccessible society, dealing with anger over injustices they face, growing up in families, living in their own bodies, discovering their identities, parenting children, finding friends, and establishing support networks with other disabled women. The first book of its type, this anthology captures the excitement and the struggles of disabled women defining themselves and organizing as a minority group.
- Campling, Jo, Ed. *Images of Ourselves: Women with Disabilities Talking*. Boston: Routledge & Kegan Paul, 1981. Rich, moving stories about women with disabilities are presented in their own words. The women vary in age, disability, work, lifestyle, and politics. (available on cassette from Recording for the Blind)
- Carrillo, Ann Cupolo, Corbett, Katherine, and Lewis, Victoria. *No More Stares*. Disability Rights Education and Defense Fund, Inc., 2032 San Pablo Avenue, Berkeley, CA 94702. 1982. This book uses photographs and brief per-

sonal accounts to introduce more than 100 different
women and girls with disabilities. It shows disabled
women and girls in all aspects of their lives: on the job, at
home, in school, with children, partners, friends, co-
workers, and family. There is also an extensive annotated
list of resources on such topics as self-image, independent
living, work, and organizations relevant to the lives of disabled women. (available on cassette from DREDF)

- Saxton, Marsha, and Howe, Florence. *With Wings: An Anthology of Literature by and about Women with
  Disabilities.* New York: The Feminist Press at City
  University of New York, 1987. Short stories, poems, essays, and other literary works by thirty women writers
  with disabilities, both well known (Adrienne Rich, Nancy
  Mairs, Vassar Miller, and Alice Walker) and previously
  unpublished. The book focuses on three themes: the
  physical experience of disability; the effects of disability
  on relationships with family, friends and lovers; and the
  transcendence of societal and internal barriers about
  being female and disabled. Building on *With the Power of
  Each Breath*, this excellent collection explores some of
  the key issues, including sexuality, more fully.

For Educators, Counselors and Trainers

- Phillips, Elizabeth. *Equity Intropacket: Women and Girls
  with Disabilities.* Organization for Equal Education of the
  Sexes, Inc., 744 Carroll St., Brooklyn, N.Y. 11215,
  1986. An outstanding and comprehensive packet of
  materials which provides an overview of social, legal, and
  educational issues of disabled women and girls, class-
  room exercises, readings and lesson plans, profiles of
  multi-cultural role models, facts about specific disabilities, and an extensive bibliography. Most
  appropriate for educators on the elementary and high

school levels interested in changing attitudes and curricula around issues of disability and gender.

- Women and Disability Awareness Project. *Building Community: A Manual on Women and Disability.* Educational Equity Concepts, Inc. 114 East 32nd St., New York, N.Y. 10016, 1984. This excellent manual examines the connection between discrimination based on gender and discrimination based on disability. It contains background information on disability rights and on women and girls with disabilities; workshop formats that will allow activists, educators and staff trainers to explore disability issues in a wide variety of settings; an annotated bibliography; and selected readings. (also available on cassette and in braille from EEC)

Resources Developed by the Networking Project for Disabled Women and Girls—YWCA, New York

- *How to Set up the Networking Project: A Replication Packet.* Materials that describe how your community can set up a Networking Project, including a community advisory board, networks of disabled women and girls, networking conferences, and follow-up mentoring activities. The packet includes sample outreach letters, program agendas, and training curricula from the original project in New York City. All can be easily adapted.
- *You CAN Serve Disabled Young Women.* A set of six training modules designed to help staff at community agencies mainstream disabled young women into their settings. Topics covered include: Consciousness-Raising on Women and Disability: Personal and Professional Issues; Independent Living Issues for Disabled Young Women; Career Exploration; Sexuality Issues; and the Use of Role Models as a Programmatic Strategy. The modules are designed to be conducted in one-hour training sessions

and can be used in various combinations, depending upon the needs of the agency.

- "Networking Across the Generations: A Conference for Disabled Women and Girls." A twenty-minute videotape that offers an introduction to the Networking Project by presenting highlights from one of the New York project's first events—a Networking Conference for Disabled Women and Girls—held in November 1984. This videotape also provides an overview of some of the issues facing disabled women in our society. (closed-captioned)

- "Positive Images: Portraits of Women with Disabilities." A one-hour videotape documentary portraying three disabled women: Deidre Davis, an attorney and civil rights activist who is paraplegic; Barbara Kannapell, a psycholinguist and well known scholar and lecturer on the culture of deafness; and Carol Ann Roberson, Director of the New York City Mayor's Office for the Handicapped and mother of two teenage daughters who is quadriplegic as the result of polio. The videotape presents the women in action in all aspects of their lives: at home, at work, with friends, partners, families, and co-workers. It is designed for a broad audience: disabled girls and their parents, counselors, educators, employers, and the general public. (closed-captioned)

For more information about any of these resources, contact:

- The Networking Project for Disabled Women and Girls
  YWCA of the City of New York
  610 Lexington Avenue
  New York, NY 10022
  (212) 735-9766

ABOUT THE AUTHORS
AND PHOTOGRAPHER

Harilyn Rousso is the founder and Director of the Networking Project for Disabled Women and Girls, sponsored by the YWCA of the City of New York. She is also a psychotherapist in private practice. A social worker, educator, and disability rights activist who has cerebral palsy, she writes and lectures widely on disabled women, sexuality and disability, and the psychology of disability.

Susan Gushee O'Malley teaches English at Kingsborough Community College, which is part of the City University of New York, and is the co-author of *Moving the Mountain and Social Change* and the author of *The Courageous Turk.* She is the Editor of *Radical Teacher.*

Mary Severance worked as a Project Assistant to the Networking Project for Disabled Women and Girls from 1984 to 1987, performing a variety of editorial and administrative responsibilities. She plans to attend a doctoral program in English Literature and Women's Studies in the fall of 1988.

Flo Fox is a freelance photographer who specializes in photographs of New York City street life. She has had many one-woman shows, both local, nationally, and internationally, and has published two books of photographs, *Asphalt*

Gardens and *My True Story*. Legally blind, Flo uses a variety of techniques and devices to enable her to shoot and develop her own pictures. These include an autofocus camera, which automatically calculates aperture (the size of the opening in the lens), depth of field, speed, and light; a magnifier; and an automatic focus enlarger. She has also developed a new technique, called photo-pointilism, which imitates her own visual perception and appears in some of her photographs.